PRAISE FOR WHY DIETS A

AN IMPORTANT BOOK THAT CAN MAKE A BIG IMPACT!

So much of nutrition is based on theory or a small sample size of data.

The information in this book is rock solid … and the METHOD used to apply the theories has been field tested by many tens of thousands of people over the last 10 years, with a remarkable success rate.

I strongly suggest you read and share this book widely … and give the method a fair try for 30 days.

Dr. David Kamnitzer

A MUST READ FOR THE ENTIRE HUMAN POPULATION!

Every person should understand how & why toxins are affecting our health and lives! This book helps bring to light why such a huge percentage of the population is in pain, sick & tired & on prescription drugs, presumably "for life", not to mention overweight &/or obese. Thank You Peter for helping educate the masses of a simple solution to ill health which can get you out of the Doctors office and out enjoying life to it's fullest! It's Simple, Cleanse and Replenish your entire body at the cellular level! Release Toxins from your body…gain health, gain energy, lose weight, gain lean muscle mass, feel GREAT!!

Carol Sanders-Holbeck

One word describes this attention getting enjoyable read…the ANSWER! After trying every "name brand diet," with my wife, I now know why our goals were never met. I applaud Peter for his work in compiling this information…information invaluable to everyone. Even if you think you're in shape, this will benefit you and can be so instrumental in helping your friends, co-workers and the ones you love. I'm almost back to the old 34's I wore in college…25+ years ago.

Andrew Levy

If you have ever tried to diet you must read this book. It has alot of great tips to why our diets fail us.

Renee D. Flack

For anyone interested in what you eat, your nutrition, what you are not getting and the importance of great nutrition and detoxifying, this is a must read. It will always be in my Kindle and will use for reference any time I can :-)

Eli S. Anselmi
BOZEMAN, MT

FORMERLY FAT / TOXIC SKEPTIC NOW HEALTHY 9 YEARS & COUNTING

My Doctor recommended diet failed! Why? It lost patience with it. It cost way too much. It lacked a detox component. (That's the short list.)

Peter Greenlaw invites you to explore WHY diets fail. His decade worth of research combined with clear, simple examples provide insights on why most diets (including mine) - leave much to be desired. When I first learned of Greenlaw's solution, I balked - big time. Thankfully, I got past my ignorance. Results?

I shed 125 pounds. I maintain a healthy weight with ease thanks to this program. I saved well over $3200 in food costs in addition to professional fees (gym trainer, nutritionist, doctors) this year alone.

Skeptics? Do your research before closing your mind. You'll be delighted and surprised with your results!

Good luck on your journey to gain and maintain good health!

Souldancer "Author, Speaker, Coach"
HILO HAWAII

I lost 30 pounds with this plan. This book explains how and why you lose weight without losing muscle. I have lots more energy. Just got a new life insurance policy at a lower rate than a policy I got 8 years ago.

Ralph E. Kirkland
DECATUR, GA

THIS REVIEW IS FROM: WHY DIETS ARE FAILING US (TDOS) (KINDLE EDITION)

This book is mind blowing! For all of you out there who know we have an obesity epidemic happening... but don't know what to do or where to turn... THIS BOOK HAS THE ANSWERS! It gives you a step by step guide of what the problems are... and how to overcome them and succeed in achieving your best health EVER! Peter Greenlaw has done his homework...he's done the research, so you don't have to! It's a quick read... but this book will change your life forever!

Robin Cermak

AWESOME INFORMATION!

This book was easy to read, full of useful information and is so true. I take the products and have had amazing results. There is nothing even close to it, out there. I have been a personal trainer for 25 years, and finally, an easy, healthy and reliable book and product that work! Buy this book...change your life!

Corinne
CALGARY, AB CANADA

Peter's research is unbelieveable! My struggles with weight, energy, memory etc were constantly being misdiagnosed. I felt I was aging at a rapid speed and I couldn't slow it down no matter what I did. His explanation made so much sense, that I adopted his views and low and behold, I have lost 24lbs and 27" in 2 short months. Never has weight been released so easily! If you have struggled. If you have tried every diet. If you have watched ever morsel you ate and have exercised your butt off without results, this is the book and program for you!

Janice Wodka

So true on so many levels. I had to try for myself and am now a complete believer! More than just inches lost -- skin firmed (I'm over 50 and my daughter noticed she no longer had to retouch my photos before posting them!) Energy levels were high before and became higher but with much more focus and clarity too!

I have been in the nutrition field for 30 years and had never done a "cleanse" or "fast" day because I just couldn't handle the blood sugar dips that go with fasting and the intestinal irritations that go with a traditional cleanse. I sailed through my first 2-day cleanse with this program without ever feeling hungry or any discomfort at all! I was shocked and amazed!

Cathleen Baldwin Maggi

YOUR LIFE WILL FOREVER CHANGE IF YOU READ THIS BOOK

Awesome and fascinating. Incredible must read. I will buy more of these books and pass them out to friends, family and even strangers because we all need to know this information. Brilliant book and makes so much sense. Thank you, thank you Peter Greenlaw for writing it!

Sharon T Amadio
CHARLOTTE, NC UNITED STATES

INCREDIBLE RESULTS - FAST!

Peter Greenlaw and his cleansing program have improved my life in numerous ways. I decided to cleanse to detox and improve my health - I already was going to the gym 10-12 times per week. In my first 11 days I dropped 15 pounds and lost 2 inches off of my waist. Since then, I have dropped more weight while adding muscle mass, increasing endurance, and strength. My waste size is now identical to what it was when I graduated from high school. Furthermore, my sleep has improved while I have more energy throughout the day. The tools that I acquired and the knowledge that I gained from this program will be integral parts of my life moving forward. Now that I am feeling this much better why would I go back?

Kevin Horvath

I LOST 11LBS AND 13 +INCHES IN 11 DAYS ON THIS PROGRAM. IT REALLY WORKS AND IT IS INCREDABLE BENEFIT FOR YOUR HEALTH

I released 11 lbs and 13 inches in 11 days and I feel fabulous. It really works plus offers an incredable heath benefits. The book describes a superior nutrition support which is the basis for the program reviewed in the book. With the after effects of Obamacare on our doorsteps I have decided to make better decisions regarding my own health and not leave these decisions up to the Washington beauracrats. Stay healthy is the best decision.

Bob Congdon

GREAT INSIGHTS AND ADVICE

Never have been able to take much weight off and then KEEP it off. Following Peter's advice, I took off 25 # and 8"off my waist. Have kept it all off for over 6 months. Am thrilled with my energy, stamina, and weight loss (never to return)

Cynthia Shelton

REQUIRED READING TO BE HEALTHY

Alarming numbers of people in the Western world are overweight, even obese. Many are confused as to why -- they diet, they exercise, to little or now avail -- and increasingly desperate to improve their health and their lives. Peter Greenlaw's book explains why so many diets and exercise regimes are not working for many people, and what WILL actually work. It is a must-read for anyone who wants to be healthy and fit,

PenDell Pittman

This is the most user friendly and informative book I have had the pleasure of reading. I have been using this product for three years. When I started using the product I was 77, and felt like I was many years beyond that. Now that I am 80 I feel 20 years younger. I have all kinds of energy and am a productive member of society. God Bless you Peter Greenlaw for writing this book. Thank you.

Letitia Hartman

The book,"Why Diets Are Failing Us," I believe is the most important book you will read on health and wellness in the 21st Century. I know it certainly has been that for me. This book is a magnificent and comprehensive treatise of the two most damaging elements of our health today: toxicity and a nutritionally bankrupt food supply. Peter Greenlaw paints a very detailed and enlightening picture of just how seriously our health and wellness have been negatively impacted by these two aforementioned evils and the exact steps we must take to combat these problems and protect ourselves and our loved ones. Peter has truly created a masterpiece. This is a must read for everyone who is concerned about protecting the health and wellness of both themselves and their loved ones. Peter, thank you for this masterpiece.

Joe Porreca, D.C

GREAT BOOK - BEST SOLUTION TO WEIGHT LOSS EVER!!

This is a great read - it talks about how toxins are affecting our health and why we are so sick. The best part is about the solution they give you. Most people just talk about it but they actually tell you how to use natural food and where to get it. It's the most natural way to eat and get your health under control. This book ROCKS!! I've been using the program and lost 50 lbs -

Rita Taylor

FABULOUS BOOK! IMPORANT. A MUST READ.

This is an amazing book. Truly important to understand this if you want to stay healthy and shed some pounds. No wonder diets don't work! If diets worked they would have worked a long time ago… but we all just keep getting fatter and fatter in this country -- and this book explains the mystery of WHY! It also shows the way out… what to do and how to do it. Thanks for making this very complex dilemma very simple and understandable. It's life-changing and life-saving.

Udana Power "Udana Power"
LOS ANGELES, CA

WHY **DIETS** ARE **FAILING** US!

Why Diets Are Failing Us!

2nd Edition

Printed in the United States of America

First Printing, 2012

ISBN 978-0-9882771-2-0

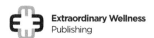

Extraordinary Wellness Publishing
#235-6834 South University Blvd
Centennial, CO 80122
The New Health Conversation Series
www.HowDietsAreFailingUs.com

The statements in this book have not been evaluated by the
Food and Drug Administration. The information in this book is
not intended to diagnose, treat, cure or prevent any disease,
nor should this information be taken as a substitute for advice
of a licensed health professional. It is always recommended
to check with your health professional before beginning any
diet, exercise or nutritional fasting program.

WHY **DIETS** ARE
FAILING US!

SECOND EDITION

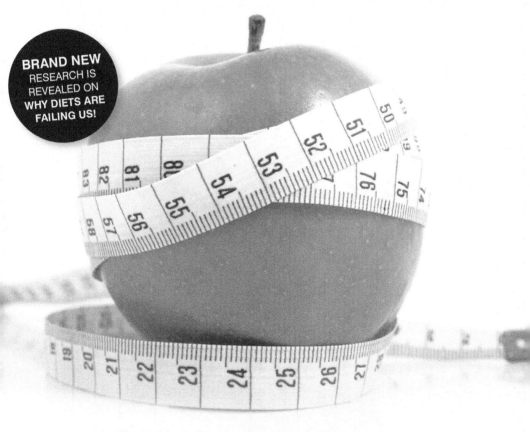

BRAND NEW
RESEARCH IS
REVEALED ON
WHY DIETS ARE
FAILING US!

THE NEW WAY TO BE HEALTHY
AND LOSE WEIGHT

BY
PETER GREENLAW, DR. DENNIS HARPER, DREW GREENLAW

Acknowledgment

I want to give my sincere thanks to the following people who without their help this book would never have been completed:

Tony and Randy Escobar, my first mentors who took me by the hand and encouraged me to continue researching, eventually leading to this book.

My co-authors: Dr. Dennis Harper, for his incredible medical knowledge and guidance, and my son Drew, who was so instrumental in completing the first and second editions of this book.

Jennifer Coulter, my wonderful editor who without her help I am not sure I ever would have finished.

My loving wife Sarah and my youngest son Colin for their love, support and belief in this book.

Peter Greenlaw
November 2014

Contents

Foreword

Peter Greenlaw has a passion for the best nutrition because he has learned the hard way when, despite his athletic background and continuing attention to good nutrition, his health gave out.

Not surprising, he learned that keeping the body healthy as we age is not as simple as it sounds in the media. Thankfully he found the right information because that is what life is about: the right information.

Everything we know we learned from someone else. Were you born into a different culture, you would speak a different language, wear different clothes, follow different customs and worship different gods. Yet they would be as true and natural and right to you as the beliefs you now hold most dear.

You have power to spare, given to you by creation as a gift right inside your genes, to develop a magnificent long and healthy life. All it takes is learning the right information to express that power. I urge you to study this book in order to achieve it.

Michael Colgan, Ph.D., April 2012
Biochemist and Physiologist Nutritionist

Preface

Most of us face a variety of challenges related to weight management, health and wellness. My own personal story is one of a dramatic turnaround in my own health almost 10 years ago. The reason I am writing this book is to share my life-changing journey and a revolutionary approach to weight management and wellness with you. It is the reason I believe that I am still on this amazing planet that we all share.

Although the title of the book, "Why Diets Are Failing Us and What You Can Do About It", suggests that I am only focusing on weight management, you'll find much more than that within these pages.

In the time since my own life-altering experience, I have helped tens of thousands of people regain their most important asset: their health. I even helped many of them achieve, for the first time, a victory in the battle against obesity once and for all. I did it by sharing this life-changing and incredible breakthrough in nutritional science in more than 1,000 lectures to audiences all around the world.

In December of 2013 it was my honor to be the keynote speaker at CEO Clubs of New York at the Harvard Club in New York City.

In May of 2014 I had the privilege to speak at the prestigious Autism One Conference in Chicago with 124 speakers from all over the world.

In 2014 my new television show The New Health Conversation began to air on PBS Rocky Mountain.

Why Diets are Failing Us has also led to television appearances for me in San Diego and in Washington DC.

It has been my privilege to conduct more than 1000 lectures all over the world on the subjects covered in this book.

Please know that I am not suggesting there is a "one size fits all" program, rather some excellent options to consider and adapt to your own body, lifestyle and personality.

There are more diet and exercise programs in the United States than ever before. Everywhere you look there are ads, commercials and articles about losing weight. According to the Center for Disease Control and Prevention (CDC), more than two thirds of Americans over age 20 are overweight, while one third are extremely overweight. It begs the question: Are diets working? If not, then what does? As a species we are not designed to be overweight, tired or unhealthy.

- Ask yourself these questions?
- Why are you dieting?
- How are you dieting?
- What if you didn't know what you think you know about diet, exercise and nutrition?
- When would you want to know?

- Tomorrow, next week, next month next year or how about now as you read this book?

The purpose of this book is to make you aware of what is available. First we wish to make you aware of the total magnitude of a problem and then make you aware of a solution that deals with the totality of a particular problem.

Why Diets are Failing Us focuses on three key principles: to live healthier, to live longer and to maximize your wellness potential. Even if you are already in great shape, I can promise you that it's in your genes to improve your overall health even further. If you have been doing the best you can based on the information you know about health, nutrition and diets but can't seem to make progress, consider that that you may be missing an important component.

This missing component we believe is to make you aware of what is now available and why what you thought you knew is not working effectively.

One of the most important reasons that diets and exercise don't work as well as they have in the past is because our world has become more polluted. For example, even if you consume adequate servings of fruits and vegetables on a daily basis, you are still ingesting significant amounts of various chemicals. Every day we are exposed to chemicals from industrial waste, vehicle exhaust, food packaging, chemically treated water, pesticides, household cleaners, plastics and more.

There is now overwhelming evidence from the National Human Adipose Tissue Survey (EPA, 1990) that demonstrates that toxins are being stored in our fat tissue at a rapid rate. Sadly, they can also be passed on to the next generation as demonstrated by studies on umbilical cords of newborns. The placenta acts as an osmotic pump to deliver nutrients to the fetus from the mother. Now, we find this osmotic pump is carrying toxins and impurities, as well.

In a study of umbilical cord blood of newborn babies, up to 287 toxic chemicals were noted in the umbilical cord blood (Houlihan, Kropp, Wiles, Gray, & Campbell, 2005). If babies have this amount of toxic chemicals in their bodies at birth, imagine how many we must have in our adipose fat tissue that is accumulating each and every day as adults.

Many of these chemicals are included under the umbrella term chronic "obesogens." These obesogens disrupt normal metabolism and contribute to obesity (Grun & Blumberg, 2006).

The American Society of Endocrinologists suggests that obesogens (Grun & Blumberg, 2006) are a major contributing factor in the dramatic increase of failing health and the epidemic of obesity. The term "obesogen" was first used by Felix Grun and Bruce Blumberg of the University of California, Irvine to explain how toxins change the way our metabolisms work and contribute to the overweight epidemic, poor health and limit our ability to maximize our wellness potential. Conventional diets simply do not offer any protection against obesogens. That is why diets are failing us. Diets simply fail in this polluted world. Healthy eating and exercising are no longer enough to avoid the toxins that are entering our bodies with the foods we eat, the air we breathe and the water we drink.

What can we do to reduce our toxic load and our waistlines? The first step is to commit to becoming responsible for our own health and safety. We have one body to last us a lifetime; there are no spares.

I want to share a centuries old revolutionary approach that changed my life and many others lives. This approach gave me real hope to win the battle against being overweight and also proved to me that it was possible to maximize my wellness potential at the same time. It is possible to release excess fat and keep it off while experiencing tremendous improvements in energy and overall feelings about life. I know because I've been there.

In this book I'll share with you the story of my health challenges and how I overcame them. I'll also give you information that will show you how and why conventional diets don't work in the long term. The scientific information is offered to you so you can understand the mechanisms in the body that create ill health and obesity. I will also offer you several new revolutionary nutritional approaches toward achieving a healthier lifestyle and maximizing your wellness potential. No not the same old approach of reducing calories and exercise as a way to lose weight and keep it off. This is truly revolutionary and highly effective in a much shorter time period than any diet or exercise program you have ever tried.

Imagine losing weight so quickly and safely that you will think your scale may be broken?

At the end of the book, I will tell you about a free support system with qualified solution advisors and a program to ensure you have multiple solutions to fit your individual goals.

Whether you have 10 or 100 pounds to lose, or you are an athlete wanting to greatly increase the effectiveness of your workouts, or maybe you want more energy and less stress in your daily life, there is a program to fit your individual needs. This program's motto is "progress, not perfection." The path toward a maximizing the most-healthy lifestyle possible must be taken one step at a time and even the smallest steps and lifestyle changes can lead to vast improvements in your wellness potential and the ability to live healthier longer.

I invite you to consider the information presented in this book and make your own decisions. If you choose to take on the challenges and techniques in this book, and do what is recommended, you will increase the odds of living healthier longer and also maximize your human potential. This book will help you decide if this program is for you, because only you can make the changes needed to live a healthier and more fulfilling life.

Wishing you vibrant health!

Peter Greenlaw
November 2014

Chapter 1
My Story

Today, I am strong, healthy and energetic, but I wasn't always like that. I had severe medical challenges that rocked me to my core and changed my life forever.

My story starts with what I thought was a routine analysis of my yearly physical lab results more than nine years ago. It turned out that there was nothing routine about what my doctor was sharing with me. I thought, "This cannot be possible." The previous year everything was normal. There had to be a mistake.

I was about to learn there was no mistake. I felt myself literally shaking inside as my doctor went over the lab reports. Fear, anxiety and so many other emotions flooded me at that moment. My whole world was turned into an unbelievable nightmare in just five minutes in my doctor's office. What was I going to do?

My doctor's stern and scary advice was to lose 40 pounds, go on a vigorous exercise and diet program and use prescription drugs to lower my cholesterol. If not, he warned, I would not have any hope to meet my grandchildren as there might not be a future. At the time in middle age that was a very scary warning. That was all the motivation I would ever need to follow his advice to the nth degree.

In my youth, I had worked out as a world-class athlete as a member of the University of Colorado Ski Team. So, when my doctor said diet and exercise were the answer, I figured I could beat this with diet, exercise, his help and prescription drugs. Despite having been extremely diligent in following a very intense workout schedule and diet regimen of about 1500 calories a day. I was very disappointed and discouraged that I only had managed to lose eight pounds after two months of suffering and following my doctor's suggestions with no cheating.

It was at that point, I was introduced to a revolutionary new nutritional approach that changed my life. I will be forever grateful to the man who discovered this new nutritional approach. The very first thing I thought as I looked at my scale was that somehow it had broken in four days. I was still skeptical but continued on.

From there, I lost 20 pounds and, to my astonishment, I went from a size 42-inch waist to a 34-inch waist, which I have maintained for the past nine years. In all, I lost over 30 pounds quickly, safely and I have managed to keep it off ever since. And, even more importantly, I continue to be free of the need for prescription drugs, which is a major triumph.

At the time, I was completely amazed but now I do not consider my story that unusual – the average weight loss for men and women is seven pounds in just 11 days based on a clinical study of this nutritional approach that I used. This still remains a remarkable feat if you have suffered through any diet and or exercise program to lose only a pound a week like I have. I was so motivated by how fast the weight came off. I had never seen anything like this before or since.

It truly can be your reason to believe that finally nutraceutical science has given us an amazing tool to rapidly get weight off or if you have not weight to lose take you to a place you might have thought was impossible.

And the best news is that for the past eleven years I have also been free of the need for prescription drugs. My story is like so many others that I have heard and witnessed over the past decade.

The transformation I saw in my life motivated me to find out why this particular program worked and why every other diet I had tried had failed me every time I tried them. It is based on real nutritional science and revolutionary new nutritional approaches developed over more than 35 years as you will discover in this book.

I believe that, if we do not embark on a revolutionary new nutritional approach to solve the overweight epidemic, there will not be enough doctors, drugs and hospitals to take care of the horrible long term negative health effects that being overweight can bring.

Our planet is changing at a rapid pace. It is well known that the only constant in life is change – happening over days, months and years. The race to become faster, stronger and smarter continues to challenge humans in every way. The advancements in technology over the past 20 years have been nothing short of remarkable yet the paradox is that technology and our constant quest to speed up everyday activities has caused the overall health of our country to decline. Some people have recognized this and formed groups like Slow Food; a non-profit association formed to counter the rise of fast food and fast life, the disappearance of local food traditions and people's dwindling interest in the food they eat.

New information is discovered and revealed daily about the dangers of processed foods and sugar. So-called "food" is no longer perceived as a "quick fix" to accommodate a fast-paced lifestyle but now "a given" on the expressway to poor health. Yet millions of people still succumb to the lure of this damaging food.

Also, there have been more than 20 scientific studies conducted over the past 30 years that show the formerly used USDA Food Pyramid and many of the dietary guidelines we have held as scientific fact are utterly false (in 2011 the Food Pyramid was changed to Choose My Plate). In fact, these 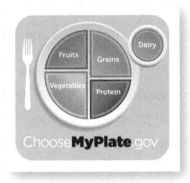 supposed truths handed down from the government are actually damaging our health and making us fat and sick. Though significant medical and technological advancements have been made in recent years, the way in which people view their diet and nutrition has not kept pace with science. Instead, we rely on outdated knowledge and techniques that do not result in achieving optimum health which is now available to everyone.

Over the last century, milestone discoveries were made about the effects of vitamins and minerals on the body. For instance, revolutionary work by Nobel Prize winning chemist Dr. Linus Pauling and his use of vitamin C opened the floodgates to understanding the beneficial effects of nutrients on the human body. Since then, products, supplements and diets have come and gone yet we still know that vitamin and minerals have positive effects on the body's overall health.

Today, there are hosts of nutritional products available: CoQ10, vitamin A, B vitamins and vitamin C along with any number of individual nutrients. Many of these nutrients have positive effects on very specific locations in the body, or facilitate specific processes, such as circulation and cell division.

There are also many techniques available, such as cleanses that eliminate the body of parasites or aim to improve organ-specific functions, such as those in the liver, colon and gall bladder. These conventional nutrient solutions and cleansing processes I call single-point-of-reference solutions.

What do I mean by single-point-of-reference solutions? What I mean is that most nutrient formulations are created to deal with a specific need or concern in the body. This structure of beliefs has not drastically advanced from those derived from Linus Pauling's original discovery of the effects of vitamin C on the body.

Considering this lack of progress we need to get back to a seemingly simple fact: the body is an immensely complex system that needs to be treated as a whole. By focusing on an individual aspect, or a singular ailment in the body, it's very likely that we are not discovering the real causes of our health issues.

Medicine is now dominated by hyper-focused specialists such as cardiologists, gastroenterologists, neurologists, dermatologists and many specialist surgeons who perform brain surgery, back surgery, heart surgery and even plastic surgery. The challenge is that each of these specialists may prescribe different drugs or combinations of drugs to deal with all of these various systems within the body. For example, a diabetic who is prescribed insulin by an endocrinologist may see a cardiologist for drugs to combat high cholesterol and may be prescribed medicine by an internist to regulate high blood pressure caused by the disease.

These various individual drugs aimed to treat a single ailment in pinpointed locations throughout the body result in complex interactions and side effects. In reinforcing or treating one organ, each of these drugs, with their own cocktail of side effects, may be damaging others. It can also be damaging to be taking pharmaceutical drugs that mask symptoms and add toxins to the body without actually addressing the underlying cause. This isn't to say that some pharmaceutical drugs aren't important but many people rely on them instead of looking at the root cause of their illnesses.

In essence, the body is a system that requires specialists to deal with all the sub-parts and specific organ systems that make up the entire human body. It is a very complicated chemical orchestration that requires special attention be given to each organ system in order for the body to function optimally as a whole.

Most importantly, beyond needing different nutrients, vitamins and major minerals, micro minerals (called trace minerals) and Ultratrace elements for each of these organ systems, the body needs water for cooling and carrying out complex neurological processes required for survival and cognitive functioning.

The human body, as a whole, is comprised of 60% water. The brain alone is 70% to 75% water and blood is 70% to 83% water. But, even after consuming a wealth of vitamins, minerals and nutrients, most people are still deficient in the simplest and most abundant nutrient on earth: water. Water, vitamins, minerals, proteins, etcetera are all vital parts of the whole. Each one is a piece of a puzzle. All puzzle pieces rely on the next to complete the entire picture. We need each individual piece but are we focusing too much on the individual pieces rather than the finished picture?

You cannot just live on one food source no matter how nutritious it is because the body requires a broad spectrum of nutrition from many food sources. For example, if one were to live on a diet of only apples, would that supply the system with all that it needs to function for long-term wellness? No. Apples are good but do not supply the body with the minimum of 51 nutrients the body requires to be nutritionally satisfied. Research says that, if you lack just one of the bare minimum of 51 nutrients, your body will never be satisfied and you will never feel full no matter how much food you eat (Stitt, 1982).

This is much like the state of nutritional science today, which has created these predominantly single-point-of-reference products to deal with a specific area of concern and not the whole system. Although some have demonstrated notable results on their specific areas of focus, single-point-of-reference solutions – to fully treat a complex system – simply do not address the big picture. This is the dilemma that faces conventional nutritional science. Having focused on improving single-point solutions for decades we have severely overlooked the real issues.

Over the past five to six decades failing health has continued to increase. Humans are in a downhill battle with our modern world and a new phenomenon has been introduced: "the body's toxic burden." As technology, transportation and food production have improved over the years, these advancements have come at a certain cost to the whole of human society and raise numerous questions and concerns. What are these chemicals doing to us? Why, in such an advanced society, is the general state of health in such decline?

Perhaps we need to be better educated about toxicity and nutrition. While there is a good deal of misinformation out there, many of us have adopted an "ignorance is bliss" attitude about our health. Though fast food is considered to be detrimental to our health and weight, people continue to eat it regularly, ignoring warning signs to the contrary. When we eat this way our bodies are forced to develop ways to protect itself from the toxicity and lack of nutrients in the food as well as deal with an increasingly toxic world. In order to protect our vital organs, many of the body's security systems are based on the production of fat cells. Scientists have found that the body uses fat cells, not only for storage, but also to provide extra protection from our modern world. As a result, we get fatter and fatter in an attempt to protect ourselves from our toxic world.

Most doctors, according to a recent survey, don't have the resources to deal with obesity. In a national survey of 290 primary care physicians conducted by Harris Interactive in 2009, 89% of primary care physicians believe it is their responsibility to help overweight or obese patients lose weight but 72% of those surveyed also said that no one in their practice has been trained to deal with weight-related issues. These findings and others come from research commissioned and released by the Strategies to Overcome and Prevent (STOP) Obesity Alliance. The survey reveals that most physicians don't have many of the tools they need to help people succeed in losing weight (STOP Obesity Alliance Research Team, 2010).

Recently, a study by Duke University projected that 42% of Americans may end up obese by 2030, which is up from 36% in 2010. The increase in the obesity rate would mean 32 million more obese people within two decades (Finkelstein, 2012).

There is no argument that toxicity, being overweight and stress lead to poor health and that poor health leads to accelerated aging and ultimately a shortened lifespan. There is a perpetual challenge in generating awareness and developing efficient solutions, despite the fact that being extremely overweight is known to contribute to more than 60 chronic diseases, including heart disease, Type 2 diabetes and many types of cancer. There are answers out there; it's just a matter of willingness to restructure the current belief systems about how and what to eat.

Achieving true health is all about nutritional density, nutritional calories and the balance of fats, carbohydrates and proteins. Cutting calories is no longer an efficient method when there is a foundational lack of nutrition. There are no "magic pills" that will melt the weight off without major side effects. To survive in this modern world, we all need to dedicate ourselves to learn from the past and move into the new frontier of nutritional science.

The bottom line is that we need to be educated on the real health issues we face in today's toxic world. Chemicals and pollutants are not going away, in fact, they are increasing every year. Being overweight is becoming a pandemic for which populations are largely unprepared.

As you will see, there is a real long-term solution to this seemingly insurmountable problem that has plagued and baffled even the medical communities for years and years.

I say "Over the last 11 years I have come to believe that the impossible is only impossible till it is not."

Peter Greenlaw 2014

Chapter 2

Dieting: What Works, What Doesn't

"If fat is not an insidious creeping enemy, I do not know what is."
— WILLIAM BANTING, LETTER ON CORPULENCE, ADDRESSED TO THE PUBLIC (1869)

The similarities in diets from hundreds of years ago until now are striking. Very little has changed. Over the years the word "diet" has drastically morphed. Initially, the Greek word "diatia" meant a sensible, moderate and dutiful way of living and originally had no specific reference to food, later it came to be associated with foods that are customarily eaten. Though this definition is still used, "diet" is now indicative of an all-consuming practice and desire to lose weight – an $80 billion dollar industry that, according to the National Institute of Health, fails 90% of dieters. It summons images of fat-free rice cakes, diet sodas, restrictive meals, point systems, calorie counting and deprivation. But how did the dieting craze of today first begin?

Dieting goes back at least as far as the 3rd century BC, according to Louise Foxcroft, author of *Calories & Corsets: A History of Dieting Over 2000 years*. She says that followers of the ancient Greek physician Hippocrates recommended a diet of light and emollient foods, slow running, hard work, wrestling, sea-water enemas, walking about naked and vomiting after lunch. The Greeks believed that being fat was morally and physically detrimental; the result of luxury and corruption, so food and living should be plain with nothing to unduly stir the passions or arouse the appetites. This was the first documented diet or "diatia" (Foxcroft, 2011).

After the ancient Greeks, it is believed that it wasn't until the year 1087 that dieting was mentioned again in literature. Apparently, that is when William the Conqueror had become too heavy to ride his horse so he decided that he would stop eating solid foods and only partake in a "liquid diet" that consisted only of alcohol in an attempt to lose weight. If the tale is true, this is the first recorded instance in which an individual changed his or her food intake habits to lose weight. Although it was never documented whether or not the diet worked, William later died from a horse accident, which led historians to believe that the diet was somewhat successful if he was able to ride a horse again (Gruber, 2002).

Since William's "liquid diet," thousands of other diet theories that have surfaced. For example, nearly 150 years ago, Englishman William Banting was advised by his doctor to begin journaling about his "diet" because he was not feeling healthy and noticed he had put on weight. What Banting did was not far from the principal belief in today's dieting world: cut sugars and starches from his meals and became the first to record the progress achieved by consuming a low-carbohydrate diet. He ate only protein (meat, poultry or fish) along with a combination of green vegetables and fruit. Banting lost 50 pounds in less than 12 months (Edwardes, 2003).

Remarkably, Banting's diet is almost identical to a famous diet that many people use today. This solution remains one of the foundations of our conventional diet belief system and it continues to follow the same pattern it did for Banting; average weight loss of around one pound per week.

Not long after the success of Banting's diet, companies began marketing a variety of products to promote weight loss. It was not uncommon for these products to contain laxatives, purgatives, arsenic, strychnine, thyroid hormones, amphetamines and other unsafe ingredients. Although proven dangerous, there is a surviving underground belief today that people can lose weight with these chemicals.

In 1917, the weight-loss industry began to focus on calories when Dr. Lulu Hunt Peters published *Diet and Health* (Peters, 1918). The success of her book was attributed to the concept of counting calories. It sold more than two million copies and became the first bestselling American diet book. Dr. Peters urged readers to view the calorie as a measurement and rather than judge meals by portion size.

It was recommended that the amount of calories in any given food were counted and totaled each day. She concluded that to lose weight it was important to stay under 1,200 calories a day.

Since Dr. Peters successful book, there have been hundreds of popular diets that use calorie counting as the principle method of losing weight.

There is no doubt that counting calories has worked in the past but, modern-day calories have changed because the nutrition contained in a calorie has diminished. The calories that most of us consume are just not the same from a nutritional standpoint as those calories from decades and centuries before. Though it can be argued that a high-calorie diet will cause weight gain and a low-calorie diet will lead to weight-loss, the body's health does not solely rely on this aspect of nutrition. If the body is constantly supplied with calories that have no nutritional value, the body will want to eat more, causing weight gain, obesity and disease. Therefore, how does one fully nourish the body without overloading on calories? It is possible and, to understand the solution, it is necessary to explore the calorie and common beliefs surrounding it.

Calorie Counting: Fact vs. Fiction

Counting calories is the most common diet method among the estimated millions of Americans who are on diets today. One of the greatest misconceptions about weight loss is that reducing caloric intake will permanently reduce body weight. Unfortunately, the calorie has become the weight loss measuring stick for the consumption of food and nutrition. You know the drill – people who count calories are constantly counting, reducing, restricting and rearranging – all to achieve weight loss, better health and better wellbeing. But they are missing a critical component.

A calorie is a unit of energy. In the U.S., the popular use of the term calorie actually means the kilocalorie, sometimes called the kilogram calorie, or large Calorie (equal to 1,000 calories), in measuring the calorific, heating or metabolizing value of foods. Thus, the "calories" counted for dietary reasons are in fact kilocalories. This unit of measurement is the amount of heat required to raise the temperature of one kilogram of water one degree Celsius (Encyclopædia Britannica,

2012). The amount of calories indicated for a given food expresses how much energy is supplied to the body in consuming it. Most health professionals and the general public associate calories with whatever they drink or eat. However, calories cannot be directly equated to levels of nutrition.

Conventional diet companies, books and health education are firmly based upon the concept of restricting calories as a sure way to lose weight. The problem with this is calories cannot be measured in the body, only in a laboratory setting because the human body cannot compute calories in a nutritional sense. The body can only use what's available to function as efficiently as possible.

Make Every Calorie Count

A new way of thinking is to make every calorie count instead of just counting calories. Today just counting calories is completely illogical if you ignore what is in the calories you are counting.

However, if calories were regarded as the most important form of measurement and all calories came from foods like cookies, candies, ice cream and sodas, these calories would have seriously detrimental effects on the body. Too many calories from these simple sugars contribute to obesity and diabetes, along with numerous other diseases.

If 1,200 calories a day were consumed from fruits and vegetables, versus 1,200 calories a day from cookies and candy, would there be a difference? Clearly, each diet consists of the same amount of calories, by a basic measuring standpoint, but in the long run each would result in two very different outcomes for the body. Eating only sugars and carbohydrates would lead to poor health and looming obesity. It is the composition of the food that matters, not the calorie itself. So, instead of counting calories as a means to lose weight, the levels of nutrition should be measured in each calorie we ingest.

From his book, *The New American Diet*, Stephen Perrine agrees that the emphasis on the counting of calories is not the way to go. "We have plenty of things that look like "health food," low-fat cakes, low-carb cookies, juice boxes that claim their contents are made from "real fruit." But they're not actually food" (Perrine, 2010).

He says that these processed food products are packed with empty calories, not nutrients, and they do basically one thing: make you fat. For example, after you eat a big bowl of empty calories from a cardboard box, your body is still waiting for some actual nutrients. That's why we eat again when we should be full (Perrine, 2010).

Perrine agrees with the basic premise that it is not the concept of calories that is most important but it's the nutrition in the calories we eat. We are overeating because our bodies are starved for real nutrition, meaning we eat more calories because our bodies are not satisfied with the amount of nutrition in the foods available in modern society. This implies that the focus should not be on the amount of calories consumed but on the nutritional density of those foods.

In a perfect world, food would contain at a minimum the 51 nutrients that research has said we must have in order for the body to be nutritionally satisfied. That is the minimum. And, of course, those nutrients would ideally be included in the fewest number of calories to sustain us.

According to Paul Stitt, "Calorie intake is only one part of good nutrition. Dieters especially are prone to the misconception that calories are all they need to count, so they fill their meager caloric allowance with foods that are high in processed carbohydrates and almost devoid of other essential nutrients, foods which can only aggravate their hunger yet never give their bodies what they really need. At the same time, the empty calories they eat rob their bodies of what nutrients they have stored" (Stitt, 1982).

In this day and age, calories and nutrition are not one in the same. As nutrition becomes scarce in the calories that we consume, we need to concern ourselves with the absorption of the nutrients that exist in the foods we eat. Only by achieving a balance in the nutrients absorbed into the body can the body's natural processes function normally and efficiently. Otherwise, we will continue to be overweight and undernourished.

According to some estimates there may be as many as 170 million Americans who are now overweight and nearly 34% of those are obese. The incidence of obesity in children under 14 doubles every six years and has reached epidemic proportions in the United States and a pandemic worldwide (Ogden, C.; Carroll, M., 2010).

To combat this growing health crisis, it is critical that nutrition be a part of the process. People need to refocus off of calories and look at balanced nutrition. Getting micronutrients such as vitamins and major minerals, micro minerals and Ultratrace elements into the body is the key to benefitting from what we eat.

A New Definition of Food's Job

My brilliant colleague Marco Ruggiero MD/PhD in Molecular biology states that food contains fats, carbs, proteins, vitamins and the Mineral Suites as we point out. Foods job is to transport and communicate genetic information to our genes. That is why what is in the calories (nutritional density and composition) we consume determines your feelings and your ability to maximize your wellness potential and stay healthy.

This is a completely new way of thinking about food and why what food contains is so critical to our wellbeing and longevity.

Two Final Questions on the Food You are Eating

Is your food doing something to you?

Or, more importantly, is your food doing something for you?

Is Exercise and Diet the Only Answer?

In America with over two-thirds of America overweight and more than 30% suffering from obesity it seem obvious that exercise and diets are failing us.

I have seen some estimates that say 80 to 90% of all diets are failing us. This is why so many people are disappointed and keep waiting for the "miracle diet." But almost a century of research has shown that dieting—which usually involves calorie restriction—is not the way to do that. Repeatedly, studies find that while eating less causes short-term weight-loss, a majority of people on diet plans gain most of the weight back within one year and the majority (90-95%) gain all of it back within three to five years (Mann, T. et al, 2007).

We are spending billions of dollars each year on diets that fail most of the time. The promise of weight loss is a great business where you can have a 90% failure rate and the customers keep coming! What a mess. I was certainly part of this false hope that the ads portrayed. In reality, I realized I was forcing myself to have hope because even though I had extreme motivation to lose weight and be compliant I had such limited success. I am not sure I could have continued on the diet and exercise program prescribed by my doctor even as scared as I was.

New diets keep appearing each year with fancy and creative names. Yet, after trying, the weight creeps back on and we are right back where we started: overweight and unhealthy. That is how desperate we are to attack the problems caused by overweight. The Surgeon General states that more people will die this year from being overweight than those who smoke cigarettes. About 60 conditions are made worse if you are obese, according to George Blackburn, Abraham Associate Professor of Nutrition at Harvard-affiliated Beth Israel Deaconess Medical Center. We should also remember the disaster of approved "miracle" diet drugs that ended up severely injuring and in some cases causing death to those who took them even under a doctor's supervision? Something is terribly wrong as solution after solution does not seem to get us any closer to solving this overweight and obesity epidemic.

What About Exercise?

In addition to diet, exercise is peddled as the missing link to successful weight loss. Although exercise supports overall health and wellness, I was shocked to learn that many experts say that it does not work as a lone strategy for losing weight. Maintaining an active lifestyle has proven to help people live longer and healthier, it is not the sole solution and is only part of the key to weight loss.

Exercise Does Not Help Most People Lose Weight

"Exercise does not help lose weight in most people but only helps to not gain any pounds. This is somewhat profound and makes you realize that if someone truly wants to lose weight, it is by improving the resting metabolic rate that you can hope to succeed. If toxins can (and they do) impair this process, we need to discover ways to improve that mechanism through detoxification and toxin avoidance" (Schauss, 2008).

As you know, I had a similar personal experience. After two months of killing myself in the gym with routines that most people would never attempt, I had lost only eight pounds. There was no way I would have kept up that extreme exercise routine with such little to show for it. And yet, in popular dieting programs that is hailed as a great goal.

Not for me anymore. No way no how and I am not ever going back to diet and exercise to the solution for weight loss and extreme health now that I am aware of a revolutionary new approach.

If diet and exercise are not working the way we've been taught, what is the answer?

You are about to find out as your read farther.

Chapter 3

Toxins: The Good and the Bad

The Enemy is not Calories
The Enemy is Toxins

We are continually exposed to natural toxins and synthetic chemicals every day – in the food we eat, air we breathe, water we drink and items we touch. Learning more about these harmful impurities is critical for making decisions to protect our long-term health.

Although we normally think of toxins only as synthetic chemicals, natural toxins have always been part of the environment. Many natural toxins are produced by plants, bacteria and animals as defenses to keep predators at bay. This natural arms race has produced millions of different toxins, including venoms and poisons, as a means of protecting the life of an individual species. One example of a toxin is caffeine. Plants began producing caffeine as a way to disorient insects that decided to snack on the plant (Weinberg & Bealer, 2001). Leaving them with caffeine high, the creatures eating the caffeine were more likely to forget what they ate or avoid the plant all together. It could be argued that caffeine could produce the same results in humans. In fact, NASA labs have identified caffeine as the chemical most responsible for human error (Wilkinson, 1995).

Human exposure and reaction to these natural toxins depends largely on how food is prepared. Cooking food breaks down many plant and animal (toxic) defenses. Also, the process of fermentation, in which microorganisms predigest a food to make it more edible, also acts to disintegrate them. According to Sally Fallon, author of *Nourishing Traditions*, almost all traditional societies used fermented and cultured processes to enhance the enzyme content of some foods and break down enzyme inhibitors. For example, without fermentation and cooking, grains and legumes are not easily digested (Fallon, 2001). Heat and fermentation can also make food safe by neutralizing plant toxins and destroying detrimental bacteria.

Still, the introduction of new foods and food preparation techniques throughout history has generated toxins and chemicals. For example, when heat is used to cook meat the reaction can emit its own chemicals, such as char and nitrosamines. And, while heat may break down the toxic defenses present in the food being cooked, the chemicals produced can have a carcinogenic toxic effect on the body.

Toxins are even produced within the human body from simply living day to day. Toxins may, at times, be produced to battle foreign bacteria and viruses. These can cause harm as they work to protect the body. But after their job is done, they are ultimately purified through biochemical processes.

All of these toxins are usually eliminated by the body without much adverse effect but in this modern environment pollution and food processing have increased the body's toxic burden considerably. Humans have added thousands of new chemicals that pollute the air and water and can often end up concentrated in foods. Beyond this,

CHAPTER 3 | 23

food is laden with chemicals in the form of pesticides, processing agents, hormones, antibiotics and other artificial ingredients.

According to Mark Hyman, M.D., in his book *The Ultra Mind Solution*, "The average person consumes one gallon of neurotoxic pesticides and herbicides each year by eating conventionally grown fruits and vegetables" (Hyman, 2009). By consuming any amount of conventionally grown fruits and vegetables, humans are at risk of harming their bodies. Since pesticides are neurotoxic and work by attacking insects' nervous systems it is believed that ingesting large quantities of toxic pesticides from our food and environment, we may be similarly and severely damaging our nerve processes.

Additionally, the continual flow of pollutants into water sources increases our risk of exposure to toxins as well. There are now hundreds of chemicals in municipal drinking water, including Prozac, Lipitor and many other pharmaceutical and prescription drugs that may have adverse effects on the body and its functions. As the body is endlessly exposed, these toxins can overwhelm the body's natural detoxification defenses. A slow accumulation of toxicity in the body may eventually disturb its natural processes.

Apparently, no one is immune to the onslaught of toxins. Even newborns have a toxic burden. In a 2005 study the Environmental Working Group (EWG) commissioned laboratory tests of 10 American Red Cross umbilical cord blood samples for the most extensive array of industrial chemicals, pesticides and other pollutants ever studied. The group found that the babies averaged 200 contaminants in their blood. The pollutants included mercury, fire retardants, pesticides and the Teflon® chemical PFOA. In total, the babies' blood had 287 chemicals, including 209 never before detected in cord blood (Environmental Working Group, 2005). Recent public tests conducted on adults in the industrialized world have shown that each person studied carries between 500 and 700 toxins in their bodies.

Furthermore, most of the foods available today are not designed to support the body nutritionally and the ubiquitous oversized portions only add to the toxic burden. Overly busy schedules and strenuous lifestyles have made processed foods a convenient option, which adds to our waistlines and increases the body's level of toxicity.

The human body has had to adapt over generations to remove various toxic loads. The body is equipped with powerful detoxification and cleansing systems in the liver, stomach, intestines and kidneys as means of protecting itself. The liver is the primary detoxification organ, metabolizing thousands of different chemicals that humans are exposed to daily. Much of what is eaten must pass through the liver. As the liver breaks down nutrients, it also metabolizes toxic substances. In most cases, these toxins are cleared from the blood and eliminated in bile or urine but, in other cases, can be stored in fat.

The body stores these impurities in body tissues such as fat even as polluted elements continue to enter the body. The fat cells then enlarge because of additional fat and the toxins are solubilized with the fat. According to Mark Hyman, there are two types of toxins when it comes to storage in the body. There is water soluble or fat-soluble. Water-soluble toxins will be eliminated through urine and sweat. Fat-soluble toxins will dissolve and recombine using fat (Hyman, 2009).

After extensive research in recent years, scientists have begun to realize that the long-term implications of toxins may result in drastic changes to the internal structure of the human body. The immune system is incapable of dealing with so many chemicals and latest evidence shows that toxins disrupt metabolism. When the body does not metabolize effectively, this can lead to overweightness and obesity. These chemicals are obesogens or foreign chemical compounds that disrupt normal development and balance of fat metabolism

The Endocrine Society, the largest organization of experts devoted to research on hormones and the clinical practice of endocrinology, reports that "the rise in the incidence in obesity matches the rise in the use and distribution of industrial chemicals that may be playing a role in a generation of obesity, suggesting Endocrine Disrupting Chemicals (EDCs) may be linked to this epidemic" (Perrine, 2010). Endocrine disrupting chemicals (EDCs) are a type of obesogen that is broadly defined as chemicals that can interfere with hormone action. These EDCs play havoc in our bodies in many ways. For example, it is now clear that other hormone receptor types and functions, including those involved in metabolism, obesity and brain signaling can be targets of EDCs (The Endocrine Society, 2009).

Obesogens

"Simply put, obesogens are chemicals that disrupt the function of our hormonal system, leading to weight gain and many of the diseases that curse the American populace. They enter our bodies from a variety of sources-from natural compounds found in soy products, from artificial hormones fed to our animals, from plastic pollutants in some food packaging, from chemicals added to processed foods, and from pesticides sprayed on our produce. They act in a variety of ways-mimicking human hormones such as estrogen, blocking the action of other hormones such as testosterone, and, in some cases, altering the functions of our genes and essentially programming us to gain weight" (Perrine, 2010).

Frederick vom Saal, Ph.D., curators' professor of biological science at the University of Missouri-Columbia has stated, "Obesogens are thought to act by hijacking the regulatory systems that control body weight" (vom Saal, F. et al, 2012). This presence of obesogens is the first reason that traditional dieting methods have become outdated. Never before have traditional, low-carbohydrate, low-calorie diets been forced to accommodate for this level of synthetic chemicals and the adverse effects they have on the body. The body's attempt to protect itself from the constant assault of synthetic toxins results in the production and storage fat.

Scientists have also found that low levels of certain compounds, such as bisphenol A – the building block of hard, polycarbonate plastic, including that in baby bottles – have surprising effects on cells growing in lab dishes. Usually, cells become fibroblasts that make up the body's connective tissue. However, pre-fibroblasts have the potential to become adipocytes or fat cells. These studies show that bisphenol A and some other industrial compounds pushed pre-fibroblasts to become fat cells and stimulated the proliferation of existing fat cells.

Scientist Jerry Heindel believes this has enormous implications. He says, "The fact that an environmental chemical has the potential to stimulate growth of pre-adipocytes has enormous implications. If this happened in living animals as it did in cells in lab dishes, the result would be an animal [with] the tendency to become obese." Heindel's studies also imply that a person's toxic burden can have consequences for three to four generations after the time of exposure.

"Researchers are reporting new data, both in animals and in humans, that indicate the effects of these chemicals can be seen not just in our bodies, but across three or four generations. So a pregnant woman affects her children, grandchildren, and great grandchildren" (Perrine, 2010).

Mount Sinai Medical School does First Study on Toxins in Human in 2005

The research on this generational battle is all without true regard for how the body is handling these high levels of poison. Major studies conducted by Mt. Sinai Medical School have shown that the body stores elements of pollution, acid and impurities in fat cells. In these studies, all participants tested positive for between 100 and 170 toxic chemicals in their blood and urine. None were free from some form of toxicity.

Considering all this information – the buildup of chemicals, pesticides and hormones in the body – it is heavily implied that a strong correlation exists between a person's toxic burden and the size of his or her waistline. These impurities may not only be helping the body to store fat but they are changing the body's genetic structures to self-regulate.

Slimming System Being Poisoned by Toxic Chemicals Creating Difficulty to Control Weight

Dr. Paula Baillie-Hamilton is a medical doctor and visiting fellow in occupational and environmental health at Stirling University in Scotland. She is also considered to be one of the world's leading authorities on toxic chemicals and their effects on our health. She believes that, "What appears to be happening is that our natural slimming system is being poisoned by the toxic chemicals we encounter in our everyday lives and this damage is making it increasingly difficult for our bodies to control their weight. The end result is that we gain weight in the form of fat and not muscle as chemicals tend to cause muscles to shrink and body fat to accumulate" (Baillie-Hamilton, 2005).

We Eat What They Eat

Michael Pollan, author of, *The Omnivore's Dilemma* and *In Defense of Food,* said it best when he pointed out that you are not only what you eat but, "You are what it eats too. If our beef is loaded with hormones that are designed to cause artificial weight gain, and we eat said beef... Wouldn't we be likely to gain unnatural amounts of weight too?" (Pollan, 2006). There must be a direct correlation between our weight gain and the synthetic hormones pumped into our food supplies. We may never turn into a "hot dog" but we may share the extra side of fat in that rib eye.

Due to the prevalence of pesticides, herbicides and antibiotics in food, very little of what humans eat can be fully broken down by the body. Instead these toxic elements are being stored as fat and ultimately contributing to the overall degeneration of the state of human health.

According to the FDA, there are now more than 80,000 chemicals in commercial use in this country and only 560 of those have ever been tested for human health effects. There is great concern among scientists and researchers about a new synergistic effect from the combination of all of these chemicals forming new chemical compounds within the human body and what the long-term implications might be.

It's no longer speculation that today's toxic world is taking its toll on the human body. Winning the battle against a toxic present and future for the human race is much more complex than just eating healthy foods and counting empty calories. Conventional dieting and exercise methods are, at best, helping people to maintain their weight but they are not providing the tools for permanent weight loss or vibrant health.

The first step is to become aware of the problem and avoid the chemical-laden, processed, empty-calorie foods as much as possible. Most importantly, it's critical to avoid exposure to toxins when there is a choice to do so. It is also important to consume more water and avoid beverages that dehydrate your cells. But the solution requires more than this basic understanding of the calorie as well as the effects of everyday toxins and how to eliminate them from the body. Armed with this knowledge, we can embark on a journey to find our best selves.

Chapter 4

The Introduction of T D O S Syndrome and Solution

Through the Research Done for this Book, We Stumbled on a Groundbreaking Newly Discovered Problem

It took close to seven years and countless hours of research to introduce to the world, "Why Diets are Failing Us". Had it not been for all the ideas, topics and new information introduced to us during this period of writing our first book, we would not have stumbled on a new concept so revolutionary that it has the potential to change the way we look at health, wellness and sickness in a new light. What we discovered was The T D O S Syndrome™ as well as the T D O S Solution™. Due to the nature of this book, we will only look at T D O S Syndrome and T D O S Solution in regards to its role in dieting and weight loss.

> **NOTE:** The T D O S Syndrome is not a disease and thus the T D O S Solution in no way is a cure for any disease or illness.

When looking at any technique to improve health whether it is going to the gym, visiting the doctor to get an overall health evaluation or changing your diet, the main objective is to improve your health. When it comes to a lifestyle change in order to lose weight, the first thing most people consider is a diet. If this is your story, you should ask yourself two main questions. Why am I dieting and how am I dieting? Usually, the simple answer to the first question is to lose weight. The second question certainly has a myriad of different answers ranging from exercise, calorie reduction and medication and in some drastic situations, surgery. As we have discussed, these techniques are not as effective as they once were. At the time of the conception of this book, we saw all these individual factors and realized that they were no longer as efficient as they once were, but we didn't see the big picture. This is where the introduction of The T D O S Syndrome and Solution was discovered.

T D O S Syndrome is the insidious interconnectivity of four individual co-factors that have come together to play a large role in sabotaging the body's natural ability to not only function optimally but also prevents the body from losing weight. T D O S is an acronym for: Toxicity, Deficiency (nutritional deficiency), Overweight and Stress. When these four co-factors combine, it sets off a perfect storm in the body, preventing the body from working as efficiently as possible. It inhibits anything from the body's capability of naturally detoxifying itself to shedding excess weight.

As was just described, The T D O S Syndrome combines four mortal enemies to the human body: Toxicity, Deficiency, Overweight and Stress. Each of these co-factors is potentially deadly enough on their own but the scariest part is the insidious interactions between the four that continue to get worse and sometimes can become lethal. T D O S Syndrome is a serious health issue that needs to be addressed for everyone but because this book focuses on dieting and weight loss specifically, let's look at how T D O S Syndrome plays a role in preventing people from properly losing weight.

Since T D O S Syndrome is a collaborative problem, we can look at it two ways. First, we can look at how each co-factor builds on each other and its power to magnify the problems. Secondly, we can pick apart each co-factor as they stand individually and see the specific effects of each one on dieting and weight loss. Initially, let's look at each co-factor as the stand-alone problems each one presents. Although this book does address this throughout these pages, we will go through a brief synopsis of these co-factors in its own little section.

Toxicity is the first of the four co-factors and plays a significant role in dieting and weight loss. As has been discussed already, the body is in a state of evolution. For centuries, humans weren't bombarded with the toxic soup that we swim through every day. The air was pure. People dealing with toxic chemicals in science labs or soldiers battling in chemical warfare areas only used gas masks or breathing filters. People would have looked at you like you had two heads if you walked down the street with an air filter mask on during a heavy pollution day. People could drink from a fresh water stream or kids playing on a hot day drank straight from the hose in the backyard. Water supplies didn't need to go through purification stations to remove sewage, chemicals and even pharmaceuticals. There was also no need to "enhance" water supplies with fluoride, etcetera. Our food supplies weren't riddled with herbicides and pesticides. Animals weren't pumped full of growth hormones and there was no need to re-enhance foods with vitamins and minerals that are now missing from our food supplies. Because of this onslaught of toxicity, the body has created obesogens as discussed. The main problem regarding weight loss is that the body refuses to release excess weight because it's a direct threat to poisoning the body with these toxins.

Deficiency, which is actually nutritional deficiency, plays a huge role on its own as discussed in the book but also as a co-factor. When the body does not receive optimal nutrition, it is obvious that it won't function at the highest level. As we already know, our food supplies no longer have sufficient levels of the vitamins and minerals needed for the body to function normally. When dieting, most approaches include some type of caloric restriction. When this is the case and calories are cut, the amount of nutrition is also drastically diminished meaning the body gets less of what it needs to function properly. The body needs proper proportions of protein, carbs, fats, etcetera as well as vitamins and minerals. When starting a program such as exercising, the body needs protein to help with both building muscle and recovery. When you combine the first two co-factors of toxicity and deficiency, you start to see how the problem increases exponentially. When the body is riddled with toxicity, it makes it harder for the body to process any nutrition and when there is a lack of nutrition to begin with, every problem is magnified.

The O in T D O S stands for overweight and this one speaks for itself. If you are overweight, there is a good chance that your body is dealing with a certain degree of toxic burden. Yes, the body holds excess fat due to poor nutrition, bad eating habits, in most cases, a lack of exercise. As you are beginning to see, it is no longer as easy to lose weight as dieting and exercise. If the body is flooded with toxins, weight loss becomes almost impossible due to the fact that the excess fat is protecting the body from itself. If the surplus of fat is released without some kind of nutritional fasting program, it is possible that it could flood the body with toxicity causing any number of problems and potentially making that individual sick. When adding overweight to both toxicity and deficiency, we begin to really see how each co-factor plays individual roles as well as the combination and it starts to look like it is virtually impossible to get healthy and lose weight.

Stress is the last co-factor in the T D O S Syndrome and there is not much to say that we don't already know about this deadly co-factor. It is no secret that stress is a killer on its own. People that are otherwise in good health have been decimated by this co-factor can suffer greatly from stress. Whether it's from the daily stresses of life or the actual internal stress put on the body from poor health or being overweight, stress is not to be taken lightly. As we know, external, life stresses can raise blood pressure among other things. Stress is also seen as excess weight and puts a significant amount of stress on the body. It literally "stresses" all of the body's functions from how the heart and lungs function to adding excess pressure to ankles, knees and the back. Once again, stress alone is a killer; add it to the other three co-factors and you have the perfect storm called the T D O S Syndrome.

One of the main reasons that dieting no longer works in the long run is due to The T D O S Syndrome. As we wrote the first edition of this book, we discussed all the factors individually without realizing how dangerous and detrimental to health and weight loss the collaboration of all these things were and the major damage it was causing.

We must understand the totality of the problem before we can even begin to find the solution. We were so close to putting it all together when we first released this book. The answers were all here we just failed to connect the dots until later. A perfect example of some of the problems we are faced with in the medical world actually happened to me just over a year ago. I accidently sliced my foot open with a power washer. Don't get me wrong and I promise I am not saying by any means I am a tough guy as there is some blame on my side of this story. When I cut my foot, it did not hurt all that bad so I did not take all of the proper steps that I should have, (cleaned out the cut immediately, etc.). Within 24 hours, my foot was swollen and hurt bad enough that I had trouble putting weight on it. At that time, I went to an urgent care place to see if there was anything that could be done. The doctor examined the cut and dealt with it based on what he saw. What he failed to take into account was that there was already a staph infection seeping into my blood stream causing major problems within my entire body. The doctor simply cleaned out the cut, gave me some crutches and something to help with the pain. Fortunately, I called my dad on the way home who insisted that I go to the Emergency Room to get another evaluation. This turned out to be the right call as the infection was already quite bad; I was lucky to not only save my leg from amputation but the infection could have killed me. The point of this story is that dieting is not just about losing weight. It's also not just a single solution as easy as exercise or calorie counting. T D O S Syndrome is the perfect analogy to this for overall health as well as dieting. So let's help eliminate toxicity in the body but if you are still eating nutritionally deficient food, the problem isn't solved. You can lose some weight but stress can still kill you just as fast. We have this puzzle and all the pieces are scattered. Yes, you can find a couple pieces, put them together and make out what the picture could be but it's not until you put the whole thing together that we will find all the answers.

> **NOTE:** The T D O S Syndrome (Toxicity, Deficiency, Overweight, Stress) and the T D O S Solution is the title of our new book in The New Health Conversation Series. This new book will go into great detail and specificity to point out the totality of the problem caused by the interconnectivity of the T D O S Syndrome's four co-factors and their potentially devastating combined effects. How in the world can you apply a solution to the T D O S Syndrome if you do not know it exists?
>
> Unfortunately if you think that diet and exercise are good enough against the T D O S Syndrome you may want to rethink that strategy after reading our new book T D O S Syndrome and Solution.

The T D O S Solution (which you will learn about a little later in this book) is the most effective multi-faceted approach to diminish the potentially devastating effects of the T D O S Syndrome. "Why Diets Are Failing Us" deals primarily with the O (overweight) in the T D O S Syndrome. The T D O S Solution book effectively deals with all four co-factors of the T D O S Syndrome. T D O S Solution is an in depth offensive strategy utilizing a multi-faceted approach not just to attack the O but also to undermine and diminish the impact of Toxicity, Deficiency and Stress. If you truly want to maximize your wellness potential and be on a path to living healthier longer then we invite you to read The T D O S Syndrome and Solution.

Chapter 5

High Density Nutrients and Nutritional fasting

In a perfect world, the body internally regulates every system at a high efficiency. If it needs to detoxify itself, it will. If it needs to burn off extra fat, it is designed to do so. The easiest way to burn fat is to stimulate the body's metabolism. To increase metabolism over time, the body needs highly nutritious sources of calories.

Because the body's hormonal and the natural processes have been confused by increased exposure to synthetic chemicals, artificial sweeteners and overall poor nutrition, we must change our eating habits to be healthy and maintain a reasonable body weight. Today's food largely lacks vitamins, minerals, and enzymes, which are often destroyed in food preparation. Humans are consuming more calories in order to compensate for nutritionally barren food. Therefore, reducing our caloric intake can no longer be considered a reliable way to maintain health and achieve weight loss. Even food companies that put forth "fortified "or "enriched" products often substitute synthetic chemicals for naturally occurring nutrients that are no longer abundant in most foods.

How You Lose Weight Really does Matter

Conventional dieting just does not make any sense anymore; yet, there seems to be a new diet every week encouraging people to reduce calories to reduce their waistlines. However, reduced calories lead to a further reduction in nutrients, thus less protection against toxins and worsened health.

Our Food Supply is Becoming More and More Nutritionally Bankrupt

The scientists are now concluding that so much of our food supply is becoming almost nutritionally bankrupt. This covers a wide array of fruits and vegetables where some of the nutrients are almost non-existent. This gets back to the whole idea of a calorie without nutrition is basically like eating air. This is why many people experience hunger after consuming huge quantities of nutritionally bankrupt processed foods. And we wonder why we keep eating and eating. Well it is because our body is still looking for the nutrition that continues to vanish.

In the book *Beating the Food Giants*, biochemist Paul A. Stitt provides evidence that supports the premise that calories should not be the standard by which we base our eating, health, and longevity.

Not Getting 51 Essential Nutrients We Need

"The organ that controls our cravings for food is called the appestat. It is located at the base of the brain, possibly in the hypothalamus (an area of the pituitary gland). The appestat is constantly monitoring the blood for nutrient content. Only when 51 nutrients are present at their proper levels will the individual feel entirely full and satisfied. If any one nutrient is missing, the individual feels hungry" (Stitt, 1982).

He continues with more scientific evidence about nutritional deficiencies effect on hunger.

In an extensive study on dietary relationships conducted by nutritionists Drs. R.A. Harte and B. Chow discovered that the absence of a single essential vitamin, mineral, amino acid or fatty acid could create a "shock wave" that hinders the metabolization of all other nutrients (Stitt, 1982).

Dieting by Reducing Calories and Ignoring Nutritional Density is a Flawed Strategy

It is clear that getting an improper nutrient balance can be almost as bad as getting no nutrients at all. It is important to remember that the body's hunger mechanism is affected by the presence of nutrients, not just calories. Although much more complex, the body works synergistically like a car. A car can have a perfectly tuned engine but, without gasoline, it won't run. Or a car can have a full tank of gasoline but the battery is dead. A car can have gasoline and a new battery however, if it has a flat tire, it is not going very far. This is how the body works as system. All the systems need to be functioning if we are to ever have optimal health and to be able to live healthier longer.

We Need a New Approach to Losing Weight and Maximizing our Wellness Potential

Although there was a time and a place for conventional methods of dieting, that time has passed. Too often, we continue to try these methods over and over again, starving our bodies to lose a little weight only to gain it back in a fourth of the time it took to lose it. This is such a discouraging cycle for anyone who has experienced it. Though this propensity for weight regain often makes us feel guilty, it's very likely that the dieting techniques themselves - not our willpower - is to blame for the yo-yo weight loss and gain that is so common in this society. The truth is that those diets were based on a premise that may have worked 100 years ago but they are not equipped to deal with the increased pollution, impurities and toxins (obesogens) of today's world.

The world is inundated with overly processed food, and because of fast-paced lifestyles and poor dietary choices, we often feel cornered into eating these food products that are high in sugars and simple carbohy-drates. The body consistently burns more carbohydrates than protein

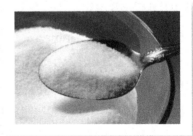

and fat for energy and this excess of sugar in many people's diets hinders the body's ability to burn off fat. It is estimated that we consumed 131.9 pounds of sugar per person per year in 2010 (USDA, 2011). In the late 1800s, it was estimated that the average person consumed only 10 pounds of sugar in a year. These statistics don't account for the consumption of simple sugars found in fruits but show comparatively that in just over a hundred years the average human's sugar consumption has multiplied by more than 13 times.

The way the body is designed to work is to burn fat, proteins and carbohydrates. During emergencies it turns to what is easily broken down which is glucose and glycogen but it will also metabolize proteins as well during this time of emergency.

We Constantly Burn Sugar Instead of Fat

According to Dr. Dennis Harper, "The problem is the majority of us are in sugar burning mode most of the time because the foods that we eat are mostly high glycemic foods that contain lots of sugar" (Harper, 2012).

Though glucose is needed in certain doses so that the brain can function properly, the brain only requires four grams of pure glucose every three hours, which is slightly less than a teaspoon. Most people far surpass this on a daily basis. The problem is that if the body is forced to consistently burn excess amounts of sugar, an incredible toll will be taken on the body's efficiency and ability to function and develop.

"As soon as the body senses higher glucose levels the insulin levels will become much higher which can result in a hypoglycemic reaction that can increase adrenaline, a stress hormone called cortisol and another hormone called ghrelin" (Harper, 2012).

What is important is that higher glucose levels cause the body to counterattack by increasing insulin. The increased insulin lowers blood sugar (glucose) and we get hungry again. It is the low blood sugar that causes these reactions to food and to carbs. We crave them when our blood sugar gets low because the brain requires four grams of sugar every three hours to function properly.

When we get low on glucose we overcompensate and we crave foods that will temporarily make us feel better but tend to be detrimental for our bodies in the long run. These high calorie foods are frequently packed with simple sugars, which further complicates the process of traditional dieting by causing the body to enter a state of stress. When we're stressed our adrenal glands respond by increasing cortisol levels, the major stress hormone. Why is this detrimental to maintaining our weight and health?

According to Dr. Harper, "Higher levels of adrenaline are necessary if you are being chased by a bear or you are under a lot of stress. Cortisol is also increased under stress to increase the amount of fuel needed for the body. It is normally produced every night to help keep inflammation down and slowly goes down during the day. Higher levels associated with stress will reduce digestion, growth, reproduction and the immune system. Sugar consumption can cause higher levels of insulin, which may produce inflammation, hypoglycemia, which then stresses the body and triggers an increase in adrenaline and cortisol, which is not desirable" (Harper, 2012).

Between an influx of the toxins and consuming a surplus of sugar, the primary systems and functions of the body can slacken and become sluggish. This reality is forcing us to search for new solutions to achieve long lasting health and weight loss, that includes being much more conscientious of the types and form of nutrients we ingest.

How Should We Eat?

If conventional dieting methods and the concept of "healthy eating" are no longer enough to maintain a healthy weight, then how should we eat? How can we be mindful and restrict caloric intake without suffering greater nutrient deficiency? How can fruits and vegetables help to detoxify the body and reach a state of optimal health while we're being exposed to obesogens in our daily lives?

The New Approach of Nutritional Density is the Key to Weight Management

First, it's important to eat in a way that focuses on nutrient density while increasing the body's detoxification potential through the ingestion of antioxidants and botanicals. The body needs vitamins, botanicals, major minerals, micro minerals (trace minerals) and Ultratrace elements as well as a certain amount of carbohydrates, fats and proteins; all of these elements are useless unless they can be efficiently absorbed into the body. Though many people are familiar with essential major-minerals like iron and calcium, micro minerals (trace minerals) and Ultratrace elements are important co-factors found in the structure of certain enzymes and are indispensable in numerous biochemical pathways. It is enzymes that will ultimately push the body to function properly and actively detoxify it. The body's ability to self-detoxify is critical for true wellness and healthy weight loss because food can be metabolized more efficiently.

The keys to activating the body's natural nutritional fasting programs are whole-body nutritional fasts—as opposed to conventional colon, liver or kidney cleanses—and being sure to ingest the needed supply of major and trace-minerals along with Ultratrace elements. Detoxifying the body is the critical key to healthy weight loss; it is the solution that delivers results that far surpass that of any popular conventional dieting program.

> **NOTE:** This is not a conventional starvation fasting approach. Do not think for one minute you will be starving yourself as that is not the case. Although this new solution (nutritional fasting) is based in part on the centuries old practice of reducing calories with intermittent fasting. This new Nutritional Fasting approach *differs in one very critical and new way.*

This new nutritional fasting approach is based on supplying the body with all the nutrients, vitamins, major minerals, macro minerals and Ultratrace elements in the fewest calories possible. It follows the new approach to making every calorie count. This new concept we call nutritional density.

The principle is caloric reduction but not nutrient reduction. This is the most important new concept in this new nutritional fasting approach.

That is why we refer to it as caloric reduction days and intermittent nutritional fasting days (very low caloric intake on a nutritional fasting day without also lowering the nutrients).

The key is this revolutionary new nutritional approach which centers on nutritional density in the fewest calories possible.

First and foremost supply the body with all the nutrients, vitamins and minerals and Ultratrace elements in the lowest calorie count. This is carried out by caloric reduction days (not nutritional reduction or starvation) with intermittent fasting days (which flood the body with all the nutrients the body needs in the fewest calories possible) this naturally allows the body to detoxify, reduce fat and shed weight quickly and safely. Yet at the same time you are not hungry because your body has a massive supply of the nutrients, vitamins, mineral, Ultratrace elements and not calories. Your body is in a state of nutritional abundance without the need for excess calories.

As you learned above if you are missing one of 51 essential nutrients no matter how much you consume in calories your body will never be fully satisfied. That is why people eat and feel like they are never full.

As you will learn we work with people who weight nearly 600 pounds and have done Nutritional Fasting without being hungry. It had nothing to do with the amount of empty food calories and everything to do with their ability to consume the nutrients they needed in the fewest calories possible. As you will learn in the next chapter as they share their amazing before and after's and incredible life changing stories.

The new nutritional fasting approach and resulting detoxification benefits are the wave of the future... and that future is now.

The Nutritional Fasting approach can put you on a rapid and safe weight loss and the path to maximizing your wellness potential and your ability to live healthier and happier longer.

It should be clear that how you are dieting really does matter.

Nutritional Fasting can give you a smaller figure but the most important reason to do it is to maximize your wellness potential and to greatly increase your odds of much longer, and healthier life.

Who doesn't want that?

Chapter 6 _____
Personal Stories

It is because of a life-changing nutritional fasting approach that I believe I am still on this planet. But it is not just what happened to me; it's what more than a million people have experienced by doing the same process I did over the past decade.

There are so many stories of people who have had incredible life changing results with this new nutritional fasting approach, it is impossible to cover all but just a few of them. These stories may not be typical, however, they are their own personal stories that I have seen first-hand.

Linda

A friend of mine had gained nearly 100 pounds **as a result of many medications** and, no matter what she did, she could not get the excess weight off. I am happy to share that she has been able to release more than 50 pounds utilizing the nutritional fasting approach and solutions. Linda is well on her way to releasing those 100 pounds so much more quickly than on any diet or exercise program she had ever tried and failed at over the last 10 years.

Mark

This is Mark's story in his own words.

"For years, my doctor encouraged me to lose weight to improve my health and wellness, but I just wasn't ready to commit to downsizing my 500 plus-pound frame.

"Struggling from a lack of energy and spending long evenings in front of the TV, it wasn't until a close friend called me and told me about this new nutritional fasting approach and solution that I began to consider making a change. I did some research, spoke with a few people who had seen results and finally talked to my wife before settling on trying the nutritional fasting.

"After using the system for only 11 days, I felt more energized and I started to see weight coming off. I knew that this new approach was what I needed to get — and stay — motivated. With the support of my wife and grown children, family members and the friend who introduced me to the program and products, I made the decision to stick with this approach for one year to see what I could accomplish.

"Now five years later and 387 pounds lighter, it wasn't the numbers on the scale that kept me going; it was the milestones along the way.

"I knew from personal experience that if I stepped on a scale regularly and wasn't at my target weight that I'd think I wasn't successful, So, I set my goals on shirt, pant and belt sizes. I have since surpassed many of my previous targets, going from a size 64 pant to a size 32. It was just awesome when I went to a store to buy my first pair of

CHAPTER 6 | 51

Wranglers in 25 years, I had to bring them back and get a pair two sizes smaller.

"My all-time favorite milestone happened six months into my weight loss journey. I was walking through a store and my doctor walked right without noticing me. I just smiled and nodded. He came back after continuing to walk two aisles over and couldn't believe it was me; he didn't recognize me. It was one of the most gratifying moments.

"That is how my journey went and I hope by sharing it with those who have this kind of weight (or any amount of weight) will see what is possible. The most important thing is that I am maintaining my weight and my life has never been better.

"My total weight lost was 387 pounds and it has been maintained for five years since the journey began."

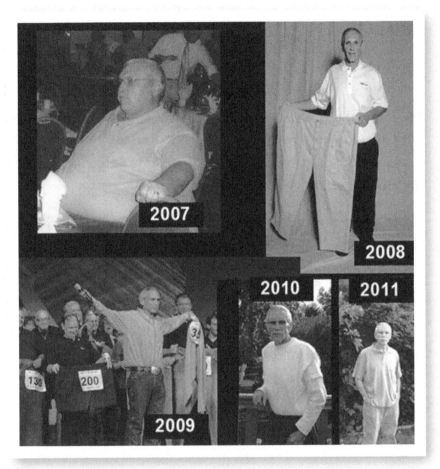

These amazing photographs show a glimpse of Mark's incredible journey. They have not been retouched or altered in any way. He transformed his body from a starting weight of 552 to 165 pounds and went from a size 64- to a 32-in. waist.

Drew and Colin

Before you think that the stories are only about weight loss I want to share one very close to my heart. It is the story of my two sons Drew and Colin. Drew my oldest son had been a member of the University of Colorado ski team and in his early twenties at time he tried this revolutionary nutritional fast. He thought he did not need to lose weight even though I assured him it was not exclusively a weight loss program.

Drew was shocked to release 15 pounds of fat, saying his energy level was that of a thirteen-year-old's. Drew has never missed a day on the program since.

My youngest son Colin was a 20-year-old all-state basketball player in great shape, or so he thought. He reluctantly went on the nutritional fast and quickly lost 10 pounds. Colin never misses a day without being on this nutritional fasting maintenance solution.

Jill

"In the 3rd grade, my school nurse put me on the scale. She told me that I was fat and weighed more than she did. In that moment, at the tender age of 8, I felt ashamed of my weight.

"Fast forward 30 years, another moment when I was swimming with my family. My kids begged me to go down the pool slide. Before I knew it, I was wedged within the slide. As minutes passed, a family member worked on getting me out. Finally, out I came, mortified.

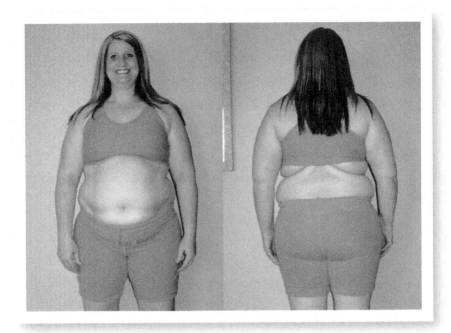

"Through the years, I've tried everything to lose weight, taking 'before' pictures 24 different times, each time saying to myself, 'this time I'll do it.' I failed every time, continuing my weight battle and food addictions.

"In April of 2010, I was desperate. I tried out for 'The Biggest Loser.' I became a semi-finalist, however, wasn't selected to appear on the show. I promised my close friend that if I wasn't selected, I would try this new approach of nutritional fasting.' With faith that God would help me conquer my addictions, I made good on my promise.

"My journey began the same time the Biggest Loser contestants went to their ranch. I made a Vision Board with the '100 Pound Club' as my main goal. I began slowly exercising and religiously following my eating plan. I was driven!"

"When the Biggest Loser finale aired, I'd achieved a higher percentage of weight loss than any of the female contestants.

"I've now released 131 pounds (half my body weight) and have gone from a size 22 to a size 4, which I also had on my Vision Board!

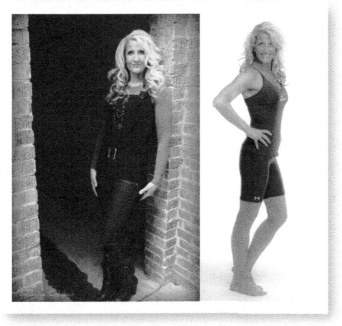

Jill lost 131 pounds!

"My new body has allowed me to accomplish things I never thought possible. For example, my son and I recently climbed to the top of a mountain near St. George. As we sat side by side on the summit, he turned to me with tears in his eyes and said, 'Mom, you did it. Thanks for getting healthy for us!' This was the same son who just a year before was embarrassed when I came to his school because someone told him he had a fat mom. Also, I recently ran three half marathon's, yet another goal on my Vision Board!

"With these priceless moments, I've realized that I will never again sit on the sidelines. I will live my healthy life to the fullest, achieving new milestones and creating new memories with my loved ones!

"I believe everyone should feel as exuberant as I do today! I've gained self-confidence and in return I'm helping thousands of people become the person God intended them to be."

Michael

Internationally renowned research scientist, Michael Colgan, Ph.D., C.C.N., discusses his own experience utilizing a super New Zealand whey protein shake and the triathletes who he trained. The following excerpts are from a lecture delivered by Dr. Colgan in 2010.

"In 1991, I wrote a book about protein, well before there was ever a nutritionally dense protein shake on the market, I wrote a book called *The Right Protein for Muscle and Strength.*

"In May of 2010, I decided to study whether or not the nutritional fasting approach and this New Zealand whey protein worked. Because there are many, many approaches out there. There are hundreds of approaches … I work with a lot of athletes. I was working with some triathletes, a group. I managed to persuade them … to do a nutritional fast for 30 days because they didn't want to lose muscle. They didn't want to reduce their food. They absolutely did not want to reduce their training. And then if their training was going to be reduced they were not going to do it … I joined this group myself because I wanted my own proof. I always want to have proof. Real solid stuff.

"So I did a nutritional fast on myself as well. And I started out at 8.95 body fat. And in 30 days I went down to 5.3% body fat. I hadn't seen my abs so well for 25 years.

"And all of the triathletes lost body fat. We lost an average of 4.9 pounds of body fat. Lost 3% of body fat. Do you think that their performance went down? No. Their performance went up. It's like taking a couple of bricks off your back."

William

My personal friend and colleague Dr. William Andrews is one of the leading geneticists in the world and has a Ph.D. in microbiology. Also, Dr. Andrews is a world-class ultra-marathon runner. Ultra-marathon runners run in races of a minimum of 100 miles continuously. That is like running four normal marathons in a row without stopping.

For years, Dr. Andrews has been researching nutrition to support his extraordinary athletic passion for marathon running which he believes is an important piece in living healthier and longer. But, even though he exercised intensely, ate three healthy organic meals a day, didn't drink alcohol nor smoke cigarettes, he could not seem to lose the extra 15 pounds stored around his middle.

That was until I introduced him to the concept of nutritional fasting. Although Dr. Andrews was skeptical about the nutritional fast, it only took him 11 days to call me and say "Peter, what the heck is in this stuff." Over the course of his first 11-day nutritional fast he had a life-changing experience. Not only did he lose some of that stubborn weight but also he was amazed (and continues to be) at the improvement in his stamina and lowered times in his ultra-marathons, which he continues to run at 62 years of age. Dr. Andrews believes that this nutritional fasting approach is the pathway to living healthier longer and is the best anti-aging strategy available today.

In August 2012, Dr. Andrews completed one of the most grueling athletic challenges on earth—a 128-mile race through the Himalayas that included two of the world's highest mountain passes. Called "La Ultra—The High," this race is run at an average altitude of 14,765 ft. and reaches up to 17,700 ft. at its highest point. Competitors have to battle with an oxygen content that is approximately 66% less than at sea level. This race pushes human endurance to the limit and redefines human body and mind capabilities.

Dr. Andrews finished the race in 5th place with a time of 50 hours, 51 minutes, 52 seconds. This feat is amazing so many ways, one of which is the fact that his competitors ahead of him were half his age. Dr. Andrews is only one of 16 people in the world to complete the race.

Recently, Dr. Andrews lectured to a large group where he stated publicly that a nutritional fasting approach (low calories that were nutritionally dense) was a major reason why he was able to compete at the highest level despite the fact he is 60 years of age. Dr. Andrews has been consistently using the nutritional fasting approach and maintenance solution since July of 2010. As a world-class athlete, Dr. Andrews has access to any food and nutritional supplements on the planet. He said that there is nothing he has discovered that truly compares to this incredible nutritional fasting approach. So, if you are an athlete and can find something better than this program please let Dr. Andrews know.

Dr. Andrews continues to this day on a nutritional fasting maintenance solution each and every day.

When Mike started on a nutritional fasting solution and he weighed 366.2 pounds. He wore size 54 jeans and 5X t-shirt. His goal was to lose 230 pounds. He was 50 years old and lived alone when he started the program. Mike didn't get out much and his friends would find him sitting alone in his house in the dark when they would stop to visit him. He had to use a table or chair to help pull himself up from a sitting position. He said he sat around a lot because it was such a task just to walk from room to room.

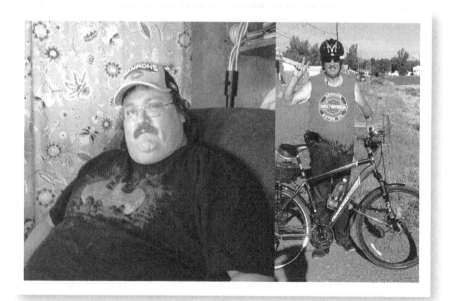

Mike now weighs 235 pounds!

During his weight-loss process, Mike charted his blood pressure, pulse and blood sugar. He also put himself on an exercise program that included riding an exercise bike and road bike.

Mike said he surprised his doctor when he saw him some time after he started the program. He weighed 396 pounds the last time the doctor saw him. When they weighed Mike this time at the doctor's office he weighed 294.8 pounds. That is more than a 100 pounds difference in weight! The doctor reviewed Mike's blood work and told him that his sugar levels were great, cholesterol was normal and blood pressure was good. He said Mike's magnesium and phosphorus and calcium was outstanding.

Mike was taking five different medications every day up to this point. Without the extra weight taking a toll on his body, Mike's doctor took him off four of his medications. He still takes thyroid medication. Mike's doctor confirmed that the key to his improved health was the weight he lost.

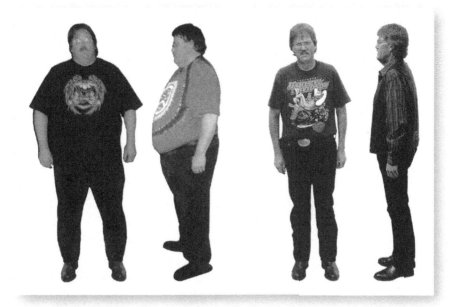

Now, Mike is active and gets out of the house regularly. He uses his exercise bike for 20 minutes every day and rides a road bike sometimes twice a day for exercise. He is always doing projects during the day whether it is working on other people's cars or projects around his house. Mike has a new lease on life. Not only does he have more energy to burn, but he says his appetite is satisfied. He also likes the fact that he doesn't crave food like he did before he started on a nutritional fasting and maintenance solution.

There are thousands of stories like these that show how people like you can lose weight, become healthier and live longer happier lives.

IMPORTANT:

If you *do not* want to learn about the solution I discovered that saved my life, please stop reading now.

–*Peter Greenlaw*

Chapter 7

What We Need and What We Don't Need

Major Minerals (macro minerals), Micro Minerals (trace Minerals), Ultratrace Elements, "The Mineral Suites"

The body must be supplied with proper nutrients for optimum functioning. One of the most important groups of nutrients are Major Minerals and Micro Minerals called Ionic trace minerals are essential inorganic elements that are required in small amounts (less than 100 milligrams) for the normal physiologic processes of the body. The body requires ionic trace minerals and Ultratrace elements to speed up detoxify and antioxidant enzyme reactions in the body. For example, selenium is needed for the production of glutathione peroxidase, zinc is essential for many enzymes and cobalt is part of vitamin B_{12}, as well as the vehicle to efficiently open cells to receive and process nutrients.

This "Mineral Suites" supports the majority of muscle functionality in the human body and is one of the key components of most body processes. While performing so many functions in the body, trace minerals also help eliminate our cravings for sugar and carbohydrates.

These little powerhouses (which make up the Mineral Suites) have been called the spark plugs of life so, when they are lacking in the foods we eat, our ability to live life to the fullest is hindered. Imagine how your car would run if just one spark plug is not working. Ultimately, our human potential is dependent upon having sufficient trace minerals in our diet.

In today's society even if a food source is organically based, it may not contain the proper amount of nutrients vitamins and this "Mineral Suites" for optimal health, our earth contains a balance of nutrients including the "Mineral Suites" for us to be healthy.

A USA today study in 2013 compared over 200 studies of the nutritional density of organic versus regular food.

Although the organic had less herbicides and pesticides from a nutritional stand point there was very little difference between organic and regular store bought food.

After many years of aggressive farming, use of pesticides, and stripping off topsoil, we have depleted the essential nutrients in our crops. A report presented to the U.S. Senate describes how diet deficiencies are related to soil depletion. The author's premise is that that the soil in the U.S. had become almost void of this "Mineral Suites" and our nation is suffering the health consequences. The catch is that the report was presented in 1936. If our food supply was nearly bankrupt of "Mineral Suites" 75 years ago, there is a good chance we have a worse situation today (Beach, 1936).

After many years of aggressive farming, use of pesticides, and stripping off topsoil, we have depleted the essential nutrients in our crops. A report presented to the U.S. Senate describes how diet deficiencies are related to soil depletion. The author's premise is that that the soil in the U.S. had become almost void of these "Mineral Suites." As a result we are suffering the health consequences. Further this report was presented in 1936. If our food supply was nearly bankrupt of "Mineral Suites" 75 years ago, we have a worse situation today (Beach, 1936).

In fact, the following U.S. Senate report, (Document No. 264) and the 1992 Earth Summit Report show the following soil depletion levels (percentages):

North America	85%
South America	76%
Europe	72%
Asia	76%
Africa	74%
Australia	55%

Research published in the Journal of the American College of Nutrition in 2004 further shows vitamin and mineral deficiencies. This study found significant declines in the mineral and vitamin content of 43 garden crops grown in U.S. markets. As well, an investigative report published by Life Extension Foundation demonstrated that the vitamin and mineral content of several foods dropped dramatically between 1963 and 2000. For example, collard greens showed a 62% loss of vitamin C, a 41% loss of vitamin A and a 29% loss of calcium.

Potassium and magnesium were down 52% and 84% respectively. Cauliflower had lost almost one-half of its vitamin C, thiamine and riboflavin, and most of the calcium in commercial pineapples had disappeared. According to the report, when asked to explain the precipitous drop in the calcium content observed in commercial corn, the U.S. Department of Agriculture replied that the 78% loss was not significant because "no one eats corn for calcium," adding that the nutritional content of produce is not as important as appearance and yield.

It is not surprising that you have to eat eight oranges today to get the same amount of Vitamin A your grandparents got from a single orange.

As you can clearly see minerals are continuing to vanish from our soil. What is causing this dramatic decrease? Scientists all over the world believe that there are many reasons.

Herbicides and Pesticides

The use of chemicals in farming prevents crops from up taking (absorbing) even the tiny amounts of micro minerals (called trace minerals) that are now left in our soil. It is not just that major minerals, micro minerals and Ultratrace elements are vanishing from our soil it is that herbicides and pesticides greatly reduce a plants ability to absorb these minerals.

Keep in mind that Michael Pollan, author of the book, "Omnivore's Dilemma," stated that we eat whatever they eat (plant or animal). In this case we cannot eat what is not in the plant or animal. This is why mineral deficiency has made food nearly nutritionally bankrupt.

Soil is Actually Alive

Soil is really alive. it is living dirt because it contains a wide array of, fungi, bacteria, plant and animal life. Soil is in a state of constant interconnectivity and balance.

All of these organisms living in this ecosystem need many different types of major minerals (macro minerals), micro minerals (trace minerals) and Ultratrace elements, to exist so they can play their part in soil's ecosystem. Minerals are a critical part of the role plants can play in maximizing our wellness potential. As the "1936 Senate Report" said "… 99 percent of the American people are deficient in … minerals, and … a marked deficiency in any one of the more important minerals actually results in disease."

Bacteria Play a Critical Role in Plant's Ability to Absorb Minerals

There are certain bacteria whose role is to convert major minerals, micro minerals and Ultratrace elements into a chemical form so that plants can use them.

Unfortunately the use of NPK fertilizers can gradually change soil's pH towards a more acidic condition in which these bacteria are unable to live. Thus the bacteria are not able to perform their function to allow plants to absorb these extremely low levels of remaining minerals.

The Problem: The Uptake of Minerals

The use of herbicides and pesticides can also greatly reduce the uptake of trace minerals by the plants. Plants also need fungi to uptake minerals. This occurs through a process that is called mycorrhiza (this comes from Greek meaning mushroom and root). The way it works is that plant roots have tiny little hairs. Little threads called mycelia penetrate the hairs of the fungi.

Unbelievably these fungi connections can cover several acres. This allows carbohydrates to be absorbed from the plant roots. This is why and how the plants can absorb nutrients from the soil including the critically important minerals, trace minerals and Ultratrace elements from the soil.

The Problem

Plants are susceptible to various fungal diseases. Therefore, these fungal diseases have the adverse effect of decreasing crop yields. This causes the farmers to spray chemical fungicides to combat the disease. The problem is also that these fungal spays can destroy mycorrhiza fungi. This causes a dilemma because now the plants have less ability to absorb the major minerals, micro minerals and Ultratrace elements.

The use of Insecticides can further reduce the uptake (absorption) of micro minerals because they destroying enzymes that contain choline. Choline is an essential component for the absorption of magnesium.

Further Evidence of Mineral Deficiency

The following excerpt from an article on mineral deficiency called "Nutrient Depletion of our Foods" submitted to: Mr. Kevin Guest, Chief Marketing Officer USANA Health Sciences, states:

"We are made of the stuff of the earth. Consequently, if the minerals are not in the soil, they are not in the plants grown in the soil; and if they are not in the plants grown in the soil, they are not in our bodies. As such, it is not surprising that any depletion in the mineral and nutrient content of our soils reflects an increase in nutritionally related diseases in both animal and human populations."

And following is a summary of the high points of this report:

- The US is eroding its topsoil 10 times faster than it is replenishing it. At the present rates of erosion our global topsoil reserves could be gone in about 50 years.
- This rapid and dramatic erosion is being caused by wind, water and by the over stimulation of soil for higher yield of crops.
- Erosions Interconnectivity with the Creation of High Yield Crops Eliminating Minerals
- Erosion's interconnectivity with these high-yield crops causes nutrient extraction.

At the same time this insidious collaboration of erosion and high-yielding crops also depletes the soil of its alkalizing minerals (calcium, potassium and magnesium). This loss causes these minerals depletes the impact of these minerals in protecting the soils from acids the natural clay deposits I n the ground and the soil resulting in the rise in acid in the soil.

Additionally, excess watering (irrigation) with hard (alkaline) water can cause some soils to leach important minerals while accumulating others (such as calcium). The net result is that soil is so acidic it cannot maintain crop growth.

Increase Corn Bushels per Acre Yield 1930 to 1960 Devastating the Soil

Imagine in 1930 an acre of land would produce about 50 bushels of corn. By 1960, this figure had exploded to nearly 200 bushels per acre. This so strips the soil of minerals and nutrients that the soil is virtually almost dead. And without the intervention of chemicals to make up for this, almost nothing would grow. As a result are producing mountains of nutritionally bankrupt foods at the expense of our very existence and survivability as a species.

GMO's May also Lead to Nutritional Deficiency

Research from The Institute for Responsible Technology shares that GMO's also inhibit a plant's ability to efficiently uptake (absorption of nutrients) from are already depleted soils.

In March 2006 the U.N. recognized a new kind of malnutrition—a multiple micronutrient depletion. According to Catherine Bertini, Chair of the UN Standing Committee on Nutrition, those overweight are just as malnourished as the starving. In essence, it is not the quantity of food that is at issue. It is the quality.

Obese Children Malnourished

In a recent study it was discovered that many of the obese children studied were suffering from Rickets and Scurvy--diseases of malnutrition. This was not because they were not getting enough calories. They simply were starving from mineral and nutrient deficiency no matter how many empty calories from food they were ingesting.

We are not trying to scare you although it may appear that way. We simply want to make you aware of the problem. If you think that food will ever be enough again when it lacks all of these minerals think again.

The good news is that now that we have defined the magnitude of the problem we can now offer hope and a solution. The earth has given us very rich undisturbed or corrupted mineral deposits that are rich in major minerals, micro minerals and Ultratrace elements.

It is possible to re-mineralize the soil. In other words to put the minerals back in the soil is possible today but the expense is enormous.

The solution is to get you mineral supplement support that does contain the 70 major minerals, micro minerals and Ultratrace elements. The formulas that we reveal to you in this book are based on your supplying your food sources with the 70 Mineral Suites as we call them.

Bottom Line:

There is great hope for your future if you do something different and turn nutritional deficiency into nutritional abundance by adding what is missing from our food back into your diet.

Becoming Aware of Mineral Suites

These "Mineral Suites" were one of the keys for transforming my life. They were either missing from my daily food intake, or present in amounts that weren't high enough to make a difference. It wasn't until I started using nutrient-dense calories (containing all the nutrients, vitamins, botanicals and the full spectrum of "The Mineral Suites") that were being formulated in 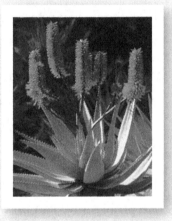 new nutritional approaches that my health began to rapidly improve.

More than 35 years ago, a U.S. patent was awarded for the extraction of these "Mineral Suites" for human consumption from ancient plant deposits that were millions of years old. It has only been in the last ten years that the total use of all these ancient "Mineral Suites" were used to create new nutritional approaches that centered on the new concept of nutritional density.

The use of these 'Mineral Suites" is one of the most critical components of nutritional density which is proving to have amazing results not just for weight loss as we pointed out. This extensive knowledge of all the nutrients, vitamins, botanicals and "Mineral Suites" that use to be in our food supply, that the concept of nutritional fasting was developed. From the first moment that I consumed massive amounts of nutrients, vitamins and "Mineral Suites" that I started replenishing these missing nutrients in my body and reduced my frequent food cravings for sugar and simple carbohydrates. It was only when I started using this nutritional fasting approach of caloric reduction and nutritional fasting that my body received appropriate life-changing elements.

This new approach can be utilized with an aloe Vera gel made from the inner heart filet of aloe Vera leaves that have been processed at low temperatures and spray dried to preserve the enzymes and nutrients. The gel is where the leaf stores the majority of its nutrients, enzymes, essential amino acids, vitamins and minerals which support digestive health and the immune system while encouraging detoxification. Also, it is the inner filet that contains special polysaccharides that have been studied for their ability to balance the immune system and their actions as natural detoxifiers (what we call toxin hunters), help move along biochemical processes in the liver to neutralize toxins. Many other Aloe vera supplements crush the leaf and the whole plant. The problem with this type of processing that includes the whole leaf is that the leaf contains an enzyme that actually destroys the polysaccharides and other nutrients. So where you get your Aloe vera from really does matter.

In addition to the beneficial effects of utilizing only the inner heart filet of aloe Vera (if you choose to formulate this on your own) and the "Mineral Suites" (that should include major minerals, micro minerals and Ultratrace elements) as a drink it should also include bilberries, blueberries and raspberries; all of which serve as great sources of antioxidants and are designed to work with all other nutrients to advance the nutritional fasting processes.

These nutritionally dense ingredients treat the body as a whole supplying it with massive amounts of nutrients, vitamins and the all so critical "Mineral Suites". Now, my body performs the way it was designed and self-regulates to achieve optimal health.

Protein is Another Critical Component of a Nutritional Fasting Approach

Half the dry weight of your body is protein; more than 300,000 different proteins. And all of them have to be made from the proteins that you eat. If you eat inferior proteins you will grow an inferior body, no matter what else you do to guard your health. If you eat inferior proteins even for one 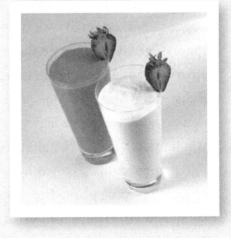 day, they will grow into your body. You will then have to deal with them for the next six months, about the time that a muscle or organ cell lasts before replacement. If you eat that triple burger, it will grow into your muscles, your heart and your brain.

To have a healthy body you have to get the right protein every day. Why is this so critical for your body? Because, the human body does not store protein but it does store fats and carbohydrates therefore if you do not supply your body daily with the best possible protein you are short changing your body every day.

Would it surprise you to know that there is another critical reason why we need the highest quality natural source of protein every day of our lives?

According to Marco Ruggiero MD/PhD in Molecular Biology, professor at the University of Florence in experimental Oncology and is recognized as one of the lead researchers in the world on our immune system. Dr. Ruggiero has published over 150 scientific papers in major peer reviewed journals on topics as diverse as Autism, Cancer and the critical role Macrophages (the main soldiers of our immune system).

This paper he published on Macrophages in the prestigious journal Nutrients

Novel role for a Major Component of the Vitamin D Axis: Vitamin D Binding Protein-Derived Macrophage Activating Factor Induces Human Breast Cancer Cell Apoptosis through Stimulation of Macrophages.

Nutrients 2013, 5, 2577-2589; doi:10.3390/nu5072577 www.mdpi.com/journal/nutrients

This paper on Macrophages is in the top 5% of all scientific published papers in history up to this time.

That is why he is considered one of the world's experts on the role of Macrophages and their critical role in supporting the immune system.

He has stated that "the food" for our Macrophages is protein.

Dr. Ruggiero, a leading authority on the immune, has stated publicly, over and over again, that this undenatured whey Protein from New Zealand is the best source of protein in the world.

This is the same New Zealand whey protein that we recommend as the cornerstone of the T D O S Solution's nutritional fasting approach.

The doctor has also stated that the very first thing he does in his clinics in Europe is a two-to-three hour evaluation of a patient's nutrition and diet.

Dr. Ruggiero also believes that nutritional abundance utilizing, this high quality undenatured whey protein from New Zealand, Mineral Suites, and amino acids have helped to improve the quality of life for even his chronically-ill patients. He says that nutrition is the key to assisting the marvels of modern medicine for better patient outcomes.

- Dr. Ruggiero asks the following questions:
- Why wouldn't you want to feed your Macrophages the best protein source in the world?

- Don't you want to maximize the effectiveness of your Macrophages?
- What are you feeding your Macrophages today?

Your very health and longevity may depend on it.

During my nutritional fast, I drank a whey protein-based meal replacement rich in essential branched-chain amino acids to satisfy my body faster and trigger muscle synthesis[1].

Whey Protein's Critical Role in Weight Management

What is whey protein's critical role to our weight management, longevity, wellness and our very existence in the toxic world we live in today? The whey protein in these "super shakes" is in a class by itself when compared to other sources of protein like meat, eggs, fish, soy and many other sources. The right whey protein has very unique properties, some of which mimic mother's breast milk: humanity's first perfect food.

The whey Shakes use extraordinary and uncommon New Zealand undenatured whey protein that can change the quality of your life and give you the ability to enhance your wellness potential and, specifically, your gene potential. Consuming these shakes provides me with incredible health benefits and energy that I am unable to get from other foods or protein sources.

---

1 To learn more about these New Zealand shakes, see Chapter 8—The Recipe, for New Zealand Super Shakes at a Glance.

New Zealand Whey Protein Mimics Mother's Breast Milk

These super food shakes utilize New Zealand whey protein and mimic the ratio of whey protein and milk protein found in mother's breast milk, which is 60% whey protein and 40% milk protein. Comparatively, regular cow's milk is 20% whey protein and 80% milk protein. In addition to whey protein, levels of milk protein are necessary while the body detoxifies itself. These two milk proteins are both excellent sources of all the essential amino acids but they differ in one important aspect—whey is a fast-digesting protein and milk protein is a slow-digesting protein to keep amino acid levels in the blood steady over a longer period of time and promote optimal muscle growth (Dangin, M. et al, 2001).

I consumed protein shakes as an athlete all my life and now I know that not all whey protein shakes are created equally. The whey protein found in this shake is derived from New Zealand dairy cows. In New Zealand, cattle are not treated with antibiotics or growth hormones and their food sources are not riddled with herbicides and pesticides. In addition, the cows are only fed grass, not corn, which is a critical component, as you will learn.

> **NOTE:** If you are a vegan there is now a vegan alternative super food shake. Eleven years ago vegan protein shakes did not contain the same amino acid profiles as whey protein. This was due to the fact that vegan shakes relied primarily on one source of protein from peas. You may also source an undenatured whey protein from Australia as well as long as you add to it what we have recommended for the New Zealand Whey Protein shakes.

In the last few years nutraceutical science has developed vegan shakes that combine several vegetable sources to mimic the amino acid profiles of whey protein shakes. We outlined what needs to be in these super food vegan shakes early in the book.

Glutathione

The amazing New Zealand whey protein in these shakes is produced using a low-temperature, ultra-fine filtering process to keep the protein folds intact. In the United States, the majority of protein is processed using high-heat pasteurization that denatures protein, ultimately altering and destroying protein folds. Particularly, this high-heat process can compromise levels of cystine, a crucial rate-limiting amino acid precursor needed to create a powerful antioxidant and major detoxification agent called glutathione. Glutathione is a substance that is critical for detoxification within the liver and in every cell in the body. Its production depends on the availability of several amino acids, along with available iron and an important trace mineral called selenium. This forms the enzyme glutathione peroxidase, which is a step in glutathione production and metabolism.

When glutathione production is low, detoxification in the liver is seriously impaired. This means the body is less able to eliminate all toxic metals, many toxic chemicals and other substances such as biological toxins (Wilson, 2011).

Glutathione is needed in every cell in the body to protect the cell membranes, cell proteins and DNA; one of two primary ways to detoxify the body. Most glutathione is produced naturally in the body but the toxicity contained in most foods today destroys glutathione levels. There are supplements containing glutathione or glutathione-sparing nutrients, however these nutrient supplements can be difficult for the body to absorb and will only provide minor benefits. Increasing glutathione launches the breakdown of impurities and allows my body to rid itself of toxins in a process known as conjugation. The toxins attach to amino acids, allowing them to become water-soluble to be removed safely through the kidneys and liver.

I had never heard of glutathione and now I understand why my health so drastically improved with these nutritional fasting approaches utilizing amazing super calories containing dense nutrition. The great news is that these unique New Zealand super whey protein shakes have all of the naturally occurring ingredients shown to significantly boost glutathione levels in the body.

Many of the thousands of research studies on glutathione have discovered that undenatured whey protein source is a great way to boost glutathione levels. The New Zealand whey protein suggested in the TDOS Solution's nutritional approach is un-denatured, which means that the protein folds haven't been altered by high heat or chemicals.

Research has also shown that the trace mineral selenium also plays a huge part in boosting glutathione levels. As you learned the "Mineral Suites" major minerals, trace minerals and Ultratrace elements including selenium added to the shakes and all the other co-factors (including aloe Vera, mini meals and super vitamins that we will introduce you to later) that make up the nutritional fasting solutions.

Proteins Role in Limiting Sarcopenia's Impact on Our Health

These New Zealand whey protein shakes also include a high concentration of branched-chain amino acids which, not only help with the natural detoxification capabilities in the body but also, maintain and build lean muscle to counteract an aging process known as Sarcopenia—a process which contributes to the body's increased difficulty in holding onto muscle as it ages.

The body begins to lose about 1% of muscle mass per year after the age of 25, and this mass is often replaced with fat. Classic Sarcopenia amounts to an approximate 40% loss of muscle mass between the ages of 25 and 70, resulting in frailty and drastic changes in metabolism. These New Zealand super whey protein Shakes combat this muscle loss by supplying the body with high levels of leucine—a critical branched-chain amino acid linked with helping older individuals retain muscle and younger individuals double lean muscle development with exercise. My classic Sarcopenia symptoms were eliminated within my own body and greatly altered my course of health for the rest of my life.

Sarcopenia is an age-related loss of skeletal muscle mass and function. According to Michael Colgan, Ph.D. - who is considered one of the world's leading research scientists on protein for over 30 years - Sarcopenia can be a deadly condition. He says, "Sarcopenia includes loss of muscle quantity and quality, loss of motor neurons that enable muscles to contract, loss of strength and especially muscle power, and a steep decline in muscle repair and recovery. Also, there is a progressive increase in oxidative stress, chronic inflammation, and pain."

Colgan says that muscles supply the immune system with the glutamine required to make immune cells, so when the body loses muscle it also loses immune function. Sarcopenia is also linked to death of brain cells and loss of cognition and memory with age because of reduced muscle contraction that leads to a decline of oxygen to the brain. He also notes that being overweight can mask the appearance of Sarcopenia, which adds to the problem.

Sarcopenia was first measured accurately in 1989 and has grown to epidemic proportions in the US and Canada. In otherwise healthy people over 40, it can be as high as one in every four tested. Colgan says that researchers on aging generally agree that it is a self-inflicted outcome that is almost 100% preventable (Colgan, 2001).

Colgan believes that Sarcopenia is preventable by consuming sufficient high-quality protein to maintain lean muscle. Later in life it is most important to have the best quality protein possible, because synthesis of muscle protein becomes less efficient with age. Numerous studies, the latest just published in the *American Journal of Clinical Nutrition*, show that whey protein, similar to that found in The New Zealand super whey protein Shake, stimulates muscle protein uptake better than many other protein sources, including other shakes (Pennings, B. et al, 2011).

Research shows that for people over age 40, the Recommended Dietary Allowance for protein [0.8 grams per kilogram] may not be sufficient. A controlled study found muscle was not maintained in subjects that ate the Recommended Daily Allowances (Campbell, W. et al, 2001).

In additional to a high-quality whey protein meal supplement, it is important to include lactase and protease enzymes. Lactase breaks down the lactose, or milk sugar found in many supplements, and protease breaks down proteins into peptides and amino acids to allow for greater absorption. With this in mind, the New Zealand super whey protein shake is the foundation of this nutritional fasting approach. It is one of very few supplements with lactase and protease that is a complete, low-calorie, nutritionally dense meal replacement.

Thermogenesis and Appetite and Highly Effective Weight Loss

An important component to weight loss is thermogenesis. Thermogenesis occurs when a portion of dietary calories in excess of those required for immediate energy requirements are converted to heat rather than stored as fat. When it comes to stimulating thermogenesis and satisfying appetite, it's well known that dietary protein is king over carbohydrates and fats. Now, a new study goes even further to show that the type of protein you choose is critical.

There are two major types of milk protein: casein (usually referred to as milk protein) and whey. According to research from the Nestle Research Center in Switzerland, whey protein consumed at breakfast, lunch and dinner proved most successful than either milk protein or soy proteins for boosting fat burning and simultaneously reducing muscle loss (Acheson, K. et al, 2011).

The scientists conducted a double-blinded, randomized, place-bo-controlled study, measuring the thermic effect of meals high in whey, milk protein, or soy proteins, with a high carbohydrate meal as a control. They found that the total energy expenditure over 5.5 hours was greater after consuming the whey protein meal versus the other proteins and all were significantly higher than the high-carbohydrate meal (Acheson, K. et al, 2011).

The thermic effect of food is a measurement of the amount of energy that is required for digestion and absorption and metabolism. Put simply, the act of eating and digesting both brings in calories and burns them. Eating foods with a higher thermic effect can support weight management goals and, in the case of whey protein, even promote muscle growth.

More than just a metabolic measure, the thermic effect of foods reflects the rate that fats, proteins and carbohydrates are broken down for energy in our bodies. The researchers explained the high thermic effect of whey protein might be due to the amino acid composition. Whey is high in leucine, a branched-chain amino acid, which has been shown to stimulate muscle protein synthesis and muscle maintenance.

In addition to boosting fat burning potential, a protein-rich diet also resulted in a much lower postprandial[2] glucose response than the carbohydrate control. We all know the feeling of an afternoon crash: eyes struggling to stay open, concentration drifting to thoughts of snuggling up in bed and overall energy depletion. Glucose may be

---

2 Occurring after a meal.

the body's main fuel source but now a new study suggests that protein should be what we eat at lunch to help us stay awake and burn calories for the rest of the afternoon.

University of Cambridge researchers compared the effects of different nutrients on neurons in mouse brains. Wakefulness and calorie burning are dependent on secretion of a neuropeptide, orexin. When neurons don't secrete enough orexin, sleepiness ensues—which can lead to fewer calories burned and more weight gained over time. When the scientists measured the actions of protein (amino acids), carbohydrate (glucose) and fat (fatty acids) on the neurons, they found that the amino acids stimulated the cells to secrete orexin to a much greater extent than the other nutrients. In prior studies, the researchers found that orexin-secreting neurons are blocked by glucose. But when interactions between glucose and protein were looked at in this study, the researchers found that protein prevents glucose from blocking the orexin secretion. Lead researcher Denis Burdakov of the University of Cambridge Department of Pharmacology and Institute of Metabolic Science simply states, "Electrical impulses emitted by orexin cells stimulate wakefulness and tell the body to burn calories" (Karnani, M. et al, 2011).

This may help explain why people may feel particularly sleepy after eating meals rich in carbohydrates. Meals higher in protein and lower in total carbohydrates could help maintain alertness over the course of the day.

"What is exciting is to have a rational way to 'tune' select brain cells to be more or less active by deciding what food to eat. "Not all brain cells are simply turned on by all nutrients, dietary composition is critical," says Burdakov.

For now, research suggests that if you have a choice between jam on toast or egg whites on toast, go for the latter! Even though the two may contain the same number of calories, having a bit of protein will tell the body to burn more calories out of those consumed (Karnani, M. et al, 2011).

Whey Protein Reduces Oxidative Stress Utilizing Undenatured Whey Protein

When considering the antioxidant-boosting properties of whey protein, quality counts. There is evidence that the undenatured form of whey is superior to the denatured form.

Unlike denatured whey protein, which is broken into individual amino acids, undenatured whey protein is carefully processed so that the natural folds within the protein are maintained. Undenatured whey protein has been shown to have greater antioxidant-boosting and also immune-enhancing abilities than denatured protein.

Oxidative Stress Major Cause of Biological Aging

Oxidative stress is a major cause of biological aging and occurs when the body's antioxidant systems are overwhelmed by the amount of harmful oxidative agents. These oxidative agents cause damage to cells and are created as a result of environmental, dietary and psychological stress as well as from the normal processes of metabolism. Glutathione is an important antioxidant that guards cells from injury that contributes to aging and whey protein is a potent supplier of the building blocks of glutathione.

Whey Protein Boosts Glutathione Synthesis Which is So Important to Older People

The ability of whey protein to boost glutathione synthesis is of particular importance to older people whose ability to make glutathione decreases with age. By their sixties and seventies, some elderly people have been shown to have glutathione levels 50 percent lower than adults in their twenties and thirties. By increasing glutathione levels in older people, whey protein helps fight oxidative stress and delays the progression of cellular aging.

Bounous G, Gold P. The biological activity of undenatured dietary whey proteins: role of glutathione. Clin Invest Med. 1991;14:296-309.Good and Bad Fats

Fats usually get a bad rap because many people aren't aware that there are both good and bad fats.

Fats from animal and vegetable sources provide a concentrated source of energy in the diet; they also provide the building blocks for cell membranes and a variety of hormones and hormone-like substances. As part of a meal fats slow down absorption so we can go longer without feeling hungry. In addition, they act as carriers for important fat-soluble vitamins A, D, E and K. Dietary fats are needed for the conversion of carotene to vitamin A for mineral absorption and for a host of other processes. Many types of fats are critical for our bodies to function properly but some fats are bad for us. In order to understand which ones, we must know something about the chemistry of fats.

Fats—or lipids—are a class of organic substances that are not soluble in water. Fatty acids are the building blocks of fats, much like amino acids are the building blocks of proteins. In simple terms, fatty acids are chains of carbon atoms with hydrogen atoms filling the available bonds. (Enig, M.; Fallon, S., 1999).

Fatty acids come in different chain lengths ranging from three carbons long to 24 carbons long. These fatty acids are either "saturated" (with an adequate number of hydrogen atoms) and chemically stable or they are "unsaturated" (missing adequate hydrogens) and chemically unstable. If a fatty acid is missing two hydrogens, it is called a monounsaturated fatty acid and, in place of the two hydrogens, the adjacent carbons "double" bond to each other. If the fatty acid is missing four or six or more hydrogens, it is called a polyunsaturated fatty acid and it is even more unstable than the monounsaturated fatty acid. Because the double bonds in naturally occurring unsaturated fatty acids are curved with a "cis" configuration[3], the fatty acids cannot pack into a crystal form at normal temperatures so their presence produces liquid oil.

Saturated fatty acids have a straight configuration and pack together easily so that they form a solid or semisolid fat at room temperature. This means that they do not normally go rancid, even when heated for cooking purposes. Our bodies make saturated fatty acids from carbohydrates and they are found in animal fats and tropical oils.

Monounsaturated fatty acids have one double bond in the form of two carbon atoms double-bonded to each other and, therefore, lack two hydrogen atoms. Our bodies make monounsaturated fatty

---

3 Cis is the Latin term used in chemistry that means "on the same side." Cis configuration refers to unsaturated fatty acids that have hydrogen molecules on the same side of the carbon chain where there is a double bond.

acids from saturated fatty acids and use them in a number of ways. Monounsaturated fats have a kink or bend at the position of the double bond so that they do not pack together as easily as saturated fats and tend to be liquid at room temperature. Like saturated fats, they are relatively stable. They do not go rancid easily and hence can be used in cooking. The monounsaturated fatty acid most commonly found in our food is oleic acid, the main component of olive oil as well as the oils from almonds, pecans, cashews and avocados.

Polyunsaturated fatty acids have two or more pairs of double bonds and, therefore, lack four or more hydrogen atoms. The two polyunsaturated fatty acids found most frequently in our foods are double unsaturated linoleic acid, with two double bonds - also called omega-6 - and triple unsaturated linolenic acid, with three double bonds - also called omega-3. Our bodies cannot make these fatty acids and hence they are called "essential." We must obtain our essential fatty acids or EFAs from the foods we eat. The polyunsaturated fatty acids have kinks or turns at the position of the double bond and hence do not pack together easily. They are liquid, even when refrigerated. The unpaired electrons at the double bonds make these oils highly reactive. They go rancid easily, particularly omega-3 linolenic acid and must be treated with care. Polyunsaturated oils should never be heated or used in cooking. In nature, the polyunsaturated fatty acids are usually found in the cis form which means that both hydrogen atoms at the double bond are on the same side.

Omega-6

Problems associated with an excess of polyunsaturates are exacerbated by the fact that most polyunsaturates in commercial vegetable oils are in the form of double unsaturated omega-6 linoleic acid, with very little of vital triple unsaturated omega-3 linolenic acid. Recent research has revealed that too much omega-6 in the diet creates an imbalance that can interfere with production of important prostaglandins (Lasserre, M. et al, 1985). This disruption can result in increased tendency to form blood clots, inflammation, high blood pressure, irritation of the digestive tract, depressed immune function, sterility, cell proliferation, cancer and weight gain (Fallon, S., 1996).

Omega-3

A number of researchers have argued that along with a surfeit of omega-6 fatty acids the American diet is deficient in the more unsaturated omega-3 linolenic acid. This fatty acid is necessary for cell oxidation, for metabolizing important sulfur-containing amino acids and for maintaining proper balance in prostaglandin production. Most commercial vegetable oils contain very little omega-3 linolenic acid and large amounts of the omega-6 linoleic acid. In addition, modern agricultural and industrial practices have reduced the amount of omega-3 fatty acids in commercially available vegetables, eggs, fish and meat. For example, organic eggs from hens allowed to feed on insects and green plants can contain omega-6 and omega-3 fatty acids in the beneficial ratio of approximately one-to-one; but commercial supermarket eggs can contain as much as nineteen times more omega-6 than omega-3!

Trans Fats

Hydrogenation is the process that turns polyunsaturates, normally liquid at room temperature, into fats that are solid at room temperature—margarine and shortening. This is the process that creates Trans fats. To produce them, manufacturers begin with the cheapest oils—soy, corn, cottonseed or canola, which are already rancid from the extraction process. Then they mix them with tiny metal particles—usually nickel oxide. The oil with its nickel catalyst is then subjected to hydrogen gas in a high-pressure, high-temperature reactor. To give it a better consistency, soap-like emulsifiers and starch are squeezed into the mixture and then the oil is again subjected to high temperatures when it is steam-cleaned. This removes its unpleasant odor due to rancidity. Margarine's natural color, an unappetizing grey, is removed by bleach. Dyes and strong flavors must then be added to make it resemble butter.

When unsaturated fatty acids are altered by hydrogenation, their curved cis configuration is straightened when one hydrogen atom of the pair is moved to the other side so that the molecule has some of the physical packing properties of saturated fatty acids. This is called the trans[4] formation, rarely found in nature. It is this process that changes mostly unsaturated oil into a solid fat. The Trans fatty acids are the same length and weight as the original cis fatty acid they were formed from, and although they have the same number of carbons, hydrogens, and oxygens they are shaped differently. The problem arises when trans fatty acids are consumed from foods and they are deposited in those parts of the cell membranes that are supposed to

---

4 Trans means "across or other side," so trans fatty acid means that the carbon chain has a pair of hydrogen atoms on opposite sides linked by a double bond.

have either saturated fatty acids or cis unsaturated fatty acids; under these circumstances the trans fatty acids essentially disrupt essential functions in the body (Enig, 2000).

Most of these man-made Trans fats are toxins to the body. Altered hydrogenated fats made from vegetable oils actually block utilization of essential fatty acids, causing many deleterious effects including sexual dysfunction, increased blood cholesterol and paralysis of the immune system. Consumption of hydrogenated fats is associated with a host of other serious diseases, not only cancer but also atherosclerosis, diabetes, obesity, immune system dysfunction, low-birth-weight babies, birth defects, decreased visual acuity, sterility, difficulty in lactation and problems with bones and tendons (Enig, M., 1995).

Dr. Dennis Harper says, "Fatty foods have been maligned for many years and not for the right reasons. Most people seem to lump all fats together as though they were the same evil food that we should all avoid."

He also says that if we consume Trans fats and our body uses these Trans fats to create new cells these new cells will leak which will cause the cells to die. When cells die they can produce lipid peroxidation, which can age the body prematurely.

The only problem with healthy fats that are found in nature would be if they have been contaminated by pesticides, hormones, heavy metals or other toxic substances. If they have been contaminated then these toxins can reside in the fats and could cause cellular death. For this reason it is important to eat clean food. This generally means organic if you can find it or growing or raising it yourself, according to Dr. Harper.

Including good fats that are toxin free into your nutritional fast is much like starting a campfire. At first, only a little bit of tinder is needed for the spark to catch fire. As time goes on, the tinder burns faster, and in order to get the fire ablaze, larger logs are needed for the fire to steadily burn. Similarly, fats are necessary in some quantities if you want to continue the fat-burning processes for an extended length of time.

So, low fat diets are not what they are purported to be at all. The body needs good fats for many of its functions like making and supporting ligaments and tendons.

In the book *Why Women Need Fat,* authors William D. Lassek, M.D., and Steven J.C. Gaulin Ph.D. explain why so much of what we have been taught about food and diets by nutritional experts, and

especially our government, is false and misleading. The authors em-
phasize that the National Dietary Guidelines and its "food pyramid"
proclaims that fat—especially saturated fat—is supposed to be bad
for us, while polyunsaturated fat is thought to be better. But there are
no credible studies that show reducing total and saturated fat while
increasing polyunsaturated fat will make us healthier.

According to the authors, one review analyzed twenty-one different
studies and concluded that there was no evidence that saturated fat
in the diet increases the risk of heart attacks or strokes. (Lassek, W.;
Gaulin, S., 2012) Another review found a complete lack of scientific evidence supporting any of the current recommendations in
the U.S. Dietary Guidelines[5]. In fact, no large-scale study has ever
shown that changing fat in the diet in accordance with Dietary
Goals lowers the death rate or extends life. They maintain that the
American people began to increase our weight at the same time we
began making changes in our national diet. These changes occurred
because of flawed high-profile studies conducted by Ancel Keys[6] and
other researchers who disregarded results that didn't coincide with
their beliefs.

---

[5] Beginning in 1980, the U.S. Department of Agriculture and Department of Health and Human Services has published every five years an updated Dietary Guidelines for Americans. The
most recent one, published in December 2010, recommends reducing saturated fat intake to 7
percent of caloric intake, down from its previously recommended 10 percent.

[6] Ancel Keys, the father of K-rations for the military, published a study in 1953 that correlated
deaths from heart disease with the percentage of calories from fat in the diet. He found that
fat consumption was associated with an increased rate of death from heart disease in the
six countries that he studied. He followed this up with a more detailed Seven Country Study
published in 1970. This study led to the McGovern Report and the U.S. Dietary Guidelines. In
his Six Country Study, Ancel Keys ignored data available from 16 other countries that did not
fall in line with his desired graph. He did the same thing with his Seven Country Study by not
using data from all 22 countries. If he had used data from these other countries he could have
shown that increasing the percent of calories from fat in the diet reduces the number of deaths
from coronary heart disease.

Because of these flawed studies, Americans started reducing saturated fat in our diets. How did this change affect us? According to Lassek and Gaulin, "during the thirty years that the calorie share of fat in our diets was going down, our weights were going sharply up." Looking at the evidence, there is little to suggest that fat intake is related to weight.

Lassek and Gaulin believe that the most important change in the American diet over the past forty years has been a huge increase in the consumption of vegetable oils high in polyunsaturated fat. More than three-quarters of this vegetable oil is soybean oil (nearly 500 calories a day) which is seven times more soybean oil consumed than in the European diet and much more than any other country in the world. Most of the rest of the oil is corn oil, and we eat five times more of this than Europeans. According to Lassek and Gaulin, our appetite for soybean oil and corn directly correlates with Americans historical weight gain. They say that soybean and corn oils promote weight gain because of the very large amounts of polyunsaturated omega-6 linoleic acid that they contain.

The authors go on to say that, "more than half of the vegetable oil we consume is polyunsaturated fat, mostly omega-6 linoleic acid, the same kind of fat that was mistakenly believed to lower our cholesterol. The amount of polyunsaturated omega-6 fat in our diet has more than doubled and now supplies more than 10% of our calories. We do need some omega-6, but a diet this high in omega-6 linoleic acid is unprecedented in human existence and extremely unnatural" (Lassek, W.; Gaulin, S., 2012).

At the turn of the century, most of the fatty acids in the diet were either saturated or monounsaturated, primarily from butter, lard, tallows, coconut oil and small amounts of olive oil. Today most of the fats in the diet are polyunsaturated from vegetable oils derived mostly from soy, as well as from corn, safflower and canola.

Modern diets can contain as much as 30% of calories as polyunsaturated oils but scientific research indicates that this amount is far too high. The best evidence indicates that our intake of polyunsaturates should not be much greater than 4% of the caloric total (Lasserre, M. et al, 1985).

Excess consumption of polyunsaturated oils has been shown to contribute to a large number of disease conditions including increased cancer and heart disease (Felton, C. et al, 1994) as well as immune system dysfunction, damage to the liver, reproductive organs and lungs. There is also digestive disorders, depressed learning ability (Pinckney, E. et al, 1973), impaired growth and weight gain (Valero-Garrido, D. et al, 1990).

In addition, it is now clear that polyunsaturated oils lower our good cholesterol or HDL. Lassek and Gaulin say, "The enormous and unnatural increase in industrially produced soybean and corn oils in the American diet is what has made us fatter. In 165 countries around the world, women weigh more where there is more corn and soybean oil in the diet" (Lassek, W.; Gaulin, S., 2012).

To back up their claims Lassek and Gaulin discuss a study conducted in the late 1990s where researchers in Heidelberg, Germany studied dietary fat and weight gain in 11,000 women aged thirty-five and older for six years. The study shows that the most important single dietary factor related to women's weight gain was the amount of omega-6 linoleic acid in their diet.

Apparently, omega-6 linoleic acid itself does not appear to have any function in our bodies but it is converted into arachidonic acid. This type of omega-6 linoleic acid produces molecules called eicosanoids. Eicosanoids that are made from arachidonic acid promote the growth and development of fatty tissue and fat storage and increase inflammation. In contrast, omega-3 fats produce a type of eicosanoid that decreases fat storage and opposes inflammation, according to Lassek and Gaulin.

Omega-6 fats also play a role in creating endocannabinoids in our bodies which are natural brain compounds similar to THC, the active ingredient in marijuana. Endocannabinoids are known to play a role in numerous physiological processes including appetite stimulation, memory, and pain (National Institutes of Health, 2009). According to a study in 2011, a diet that is high in omega-6 polyunsaturated fatty acids will cause an increase in endocannabinoid signaling system activation and stimulate tissue specific activities that decrease insulin sensitivity in muscle and promote fat accumulation in the adipose tissue. (Kim,J; Li, Y; Watkins, B, 2011).

The other way the omega-6 in our diet makes us gain weight is by decreasing omega-3 in our bodies—the fat that helps makes us thinner. In the German study of dietary fat and weight gain, the more omega-3 fats in a woman's diet (alpha-linolenic, DHA, and EPA) the less weight she gained over time (Lassek, W.; Gaulin, S., 2012).

Instead of increasing fat storage and weight gain, omega-3 helps to reduce weight by increasing fat burning and decreasing the amount of fat we store. Also, omega 3 helps decrease our appetite. It is common to be hungrier after meals high in omega-6 linoleic acid and less hungry after meals high in omega-3. Omega-3 fats also help improve the way our cells respond to insulin which can improve blood sugar control.

Lassek and Gaulin say that in 1960 we consumed nine times more omega-6 than omega-3, while today we have more than 21 times as much. Making matters still worse, as our omega-6 has been increasing; we have also been getting less omega-3 from some of the natural sources of omega-3 (EPA and DHA) in our diets, in the form of meat, poultry, eggs and fish.

"The amount of omega fats in meat depends on what the animals eat. And most animals are now fed corn instead of grass because it's cheaper. Since corn is much higher in omega-6 and much lower in omega-3 than grass, the change in animal feeds has lowered the omega-3 in meat and eggs while increasing omega-6. And while chicken meat and eggs still have some omega-3 EPA and DHA they now have much more omega-6 than omega-3 because chickens have also been switched over to corn-based feed" (Lassek, W.; Gaulin, S., 2012). That is why it is so significant that The New Zealand super whey protein Shakes are made with whey protein from cows that only eat grass.

Dr. Donald Miller, a cardiac surgeon and professor of surgery at the University Of Washington School Of Medicine in Seattle, puts our nation's health crisis in perspective. He says that 100 years ago less than one in one hundred Americans were obese and coronary heart disease was unknown. Pneumonia, diarrhea and enteritis, and tuberculosis were the most common causes of death. Now, a century later, the two most common causes of death are coronary heart disease and cancer, which account for 75 percent of all deaths in this country. There were 500 cardiologists practicing in the U.S. in 1950. There are 30,000 of them now – a 60-fold increase for a population that has only doubled since 1950 (Miller, D., 2011).

He goes on to say that an epidemic of obesity has accompanied the adoption of a low-fat diet. With only 1 in 150 people obese when the century began, by 1950 nearly 10 percent of Americans were obese. Thirty years later, in 1980, it had risen to 15 percent. Then following publication of the U.S. Dietary Guidelines and its every-five-year updates, obesity in Americans has steadily risen. Now, two-thirds of the American public is overweight and more than one-third is obese. Today the average American weighs 30 pounds more that he or she did 100 years ago. American women weigh an average of 167 pounds and men weigh and average of 191 pounds.

Dr. Miller contends that, "there is solid evidence that this epidemic of obesity has resulted from replacing saturated fat in the American diet with carbohydrates and processed polyunsaturated vegetable oils" (Miller, D., 2011).

These are some of the reasons why we have become one of the most overfed and undernourished societies on earth. Look around at our obese nation. Is the Food Pyramid working? We have been flat out misled at the very least. There was never any evidence that saturated fats were bad; it is the polyunsaturated omega-6 fats that are bad while the omega-3 fats are the good guys. It's this important knowledge that can help us finding a solution to this giant problem we are having with being overweight, and why diets are failing us.

Chapter 8
The Solution

Introducing The T D O S Solution

So far, we have outlined a number of problems and reasons why diets are not and never will be enough again. The proof is out there between the food sources that no longer harbor the essential nutrients the body needs to the fact that we are unable to detoxify ourselves using the old school methods from fasting to saunas. We need a new approach as the rules have changed. This approach needs to be one based off new ideas and perceptions. It's time to view the body as a whole. Weight loss can no longer be viewed as just losing weight and the techniques can't just be targeted towards shrinking the waistline. The body is a system and it only makes sense to treat it accordingly. The example I used with my foot and the staph infection once again strengthens that argument. Yes, the external problem was the cut on my foot but the internal, systematic problem could have been life threatening.

The T D O S Syndrome was just introduced as the collaboration of four co-factors that individually are capable of causing any number of health problems but when they synthesize, the problems grow increasingly dangerous. Much in the same way we discovered The

T D O S Syndrome, we have come up with the best way to manage these problems with The T D O S Solution.

Because it took the writing of this book to put together both T D O S Syndrome and Solution, we believe that the power of both of these concepts was great enough to follow up this book with a two part book explaining in depth both T D O S Syndrome and T D O S Solution. When looking at why diets are failing us, it is now apparent that if one of the main problems of why diets fail is due to T D O S Syndrome, it only makes sense that the first solution as far as what to do to combat poor health, excess weight, stress, etcetera, is to follow the T D O S Solution.

The premise of T D O S Solution is a combative one. How can we take each co-factor and either eliminate it or reduce its grasp on our health and wellness? Some of these answers will present themselves in the remaining pages of this book. If we are capable of taking a step back and looking at the big picture, we can look at each co-factor and how to handle it properly, thus effectively and safely begin to address each issue from detoxifying, losing weight, eating a balanced diet and even lowering stress.

The T D O S Solution is an all-inclusive answer to maximizing your wellness potential through regaining optimal health on every level from maintaining a healthy weight to reduced stress both mentally and physically. Once again, T D O S Solution is about managing health as a system. We must look at the totality of the problem before finding a solution.

Unfortunately if you think that diet and exercise are good enough against the T D O S Syndrome good luck with that strategy.

The T D O S Solution is the most effective multi-faceted approach to diminish the horrible effects of the T D O S Syndrome. "Why Diets are Failing" Us deals primarily with the O in the T D O S Syndrome. The T D O S Solution effectively deals with all four co-factors of the T D O S Syndrome and is critical to maximizing your wellness potential and living healthier longer.

The Healing Practice of Nutritional Fasting

Fasting has been a traditional healing practice for thousands of years to enhance many of the body's internal detoxification and cleansing systems. Throughout history, a common method for detoxification has been fasting while only ingesting a combination of herbal teas or special botanicals. Reduced food intake allows the body to purify itself through rest and renewal, while botanicals, such as aloe gel, licorice root and ashwagandha root contain bio-active components to support the liver, the body's natural detoxifier and individual cells.

Age-old traditions of fasting have now been combined with modern technologies to new nutritional approaches that provide nourishment to efficiently deal with daily toxic loads and stresses. In my own quest to detoxify my body, I used the T D O S Solution's suggested use of an Aloe Vera juice drink utilizing the inner heart filet of the aloe plant and enhanced with the "Mineral Suites"; a drink to support the liver, immune system and overall cellular health by utilizing a combination of vitamins, herbal teas and other botanical ingredients.

How and Why the TDOS Solution's™ Nutritional Fasting Works

By now you must be wondering how the TDOS Solution's Nutritional Fasting approach works so dramatically and safely.

The TDOS Solution's nutritional fasting approach is by any conventional means not a diet that focuses on counting calories but a complete program that allows the body to naturally detoxify itself. This is the most important concept: *the body can detoxify itself by being supplied with massive amounts of nutrients in very few calories, consumed in a very specific way.*

We give you a very specific road map for how and when to consume these formulas. This is a critical component to the success of the TDOS Solution; as the implementation of the formula's combination of intermittent caloric reductions (not nutritional reductions) and 48 hour of nutritional fasting (caloric reduction not nutritional reduction) are critical.

Reducing Calories and not Reduction of Nutrients is the Key to a Nutritional Fasting Approach

NOTE: When we say caloric restriction we are not talking about nutrient restriction. As you are getting massive amounts of nutrients even when you restrict these super calories contained in the formulas we have laid out for you. Shift your thinking about counting how many calories you are consuming and instead focus on how many nutrients does my body need to function at its maximum wellness potential.

This is why the T D O S Solution's caloric restriction and intermittent fasting approach works as we have now said many times. It is so important that you realize the breakthrough that has provided so many people with the hope of finally get their weight under control and in turn the hope of maximizing their wellness potential.

The Aloe Vera Mineral Drink is Critical to Nutritional Fasting

The ingredients chosen for the aloe Vera mineral drink helped protect my body from daily pollutants and promoted a state of "deep nutritional fasting" so I could embark on a sound approach to weight management that actually works in the long term.

Balanced nutrition and nutritional fasting are key strategies for coping with daily toxins but there are others. Since there's no way to avoid all toxins and balanced nutrition and nutritional fasting are only partial strategies for coping, additional measures must be taken. The goal, of course, is to reduce toxic exposure as much as possible. I was able to achieve this by making simple lifestyle changes such as choosing fruits and vegetables free of pesticides, drinking more water, using non-toxic skin care products and being in the fresh air whenever possible.

How Does the Program Work?

The following nutritional fasting program is not a diet that focuses on counting calories but a complete program that allows the body to detoxify itself naturally. This can naturally lead to a much healthier and more vibrant life not matter if you are old or young overweight or in great shape.

It all begins with caloric reduction super food shake days (utilizing the New Zealand whey protein shakes). An advisor can help you decide based on your goals to begin with 2 to 5 days of caloric reduction (remember you are not lowering the nutrients, vitamins and Mineral Suites).

We have found that after completing you caloric reduction super shake days you do two days (48 hours) of nutritional fasting Again this is very low calories with extremely highly concentrated nutritional density. This is both why and how it works as you will learn shortly as we will lay out the nutritional fasting approach and maintenance program in this book.

During my nutritional fast, it surprised me that even on nutritional fasting days (maximum of 48 hours in a row) when I was only ingesting liquid nutrition, my body was fed and satisfied with massive amounts of liquid nutrition and though caloric intake is severely reduced, the body is not denied the important nutrients, vitamins and Minerals Suites it needed. I was pleasantly surprised that I was not hungry.

As my body was optimally supplied with the necessary nutrients without all the calories, my body naturally began to naturally detoxify by utilizing the massive amounts of these nutrients contained in this new nutritional approach that made up this life-changing nutritional fasting solution.

The "Mineral Suites" supported the enzymes naturally occurring in my body. Impurities stored in fat cells traveled to my liver to be detoxified. The liver then released these impurities as bile or converted them into water-soluble waste to be processed by my liver and excreted from my body through the colon. This process differs greatly from a colon detoxify, which is designed to release toxins only in the colon, not the toxins stored in our fat cells. I did not spend additional time in the bathroom. This is nothing like a colon detoxify, not that a colon detoxify is bad.

While I was on the T D O S Solution's nutritional fasting approach, I consumed The New Zealand super whey protein-Shakes and a series of chewable mini-meals in a wafer sized snack that are packed with the same New Zealand whey protein as in the shakes. These low-calorie nutritionally dense mini-meals helped to curb my hunger by providing small amounts of proteins, fats and carbohydrates throughout the day to keep my body in balance and prevent the oft-cited "afternoon crash" of energy. These mini-meals maintained overall balance in my body, with proteins to support lean muscle development, carbohydrates to break down into glucose to keep the brain sharp and the "Mineral Suites" to keep me fully nourished. These mini meals contain a certain amount of fats, such as organic coconut oil, needed to slow down the release of glucose, maintain my body's fat-burning processes and stimulate metabolism firings. The last component in the nutritional fast is what I like to refer to as a super vitamin. This super vitamin or unique capsule assists my body in burning fat without the use of stimulants. These capsules naturally invigorated my body to maintain energy throughout the day while on the nutritional fast. Each capsule contains the "Mineral

Suites" co-factors and a variety of natural ingredients, including apple cider vinegar, green tea leaf extract, niacin, cinnamon-dried bark and cayenne pepper.

If you want to source your own super vitamin make sure it contains all of these ingredients.

Even on nutritional fasting days, these natural vitamins, nutrients and the all-important Mineral Suites ensured that my body was constantly satisfied with pure nourishment. Keep in mind that the Super vitamin is for appetite support and not for appetite suppression.

Why Does Nutritional Fasting Produce Such Dramatic Results?

Herein lies the secret to the long-lasting success of this revolutionary nutritional fast; though low in calories, the T D O S Solution's nutritional fasting approach provided me with nutritionally dense calories. It gave me all the vitamins, nutrients and the Mineral Suites" to totally satisfy and meet the cellular requirements for maximum wellness and extremely successful long term weight loss.

As we have previously discussed, most of today's foods are not nutritionally balanced or nutritionally dense so people continue to crave and consume more and more food that never fully nourishes or satisfies them. However, the T D O S Solution nutritional fasting approaches supply massive amounts of nutrition and the critical "Mineral Suites" in very few calories.

The new nutritional fasting approach supplies the body with many more than the minimum 51 nutrients required for minimum human body functions. The "Mineral Suites" we recommend in the T D O S Solutions nutritional approach should include a combination of major minerals (macro minerals), micro minerals (trace minerals) and Ultratrace elements.

During my nutritional fasting experience, antioxidant botanicals such as aloe gel, licorice root and ashwagandha root supported liver detoxification and reduced my cravings as my body was consistently flooded with nutritious elements and the "Mineral Suites" instead of empty calories.

Even when my body was immersed in a nutritional fasting day, I was continually satisfied because for the first time I was supplied with the appropriate amounts of vitamins, nutrition, minerals and Ultratrace elements – a need that extends far beyond just calories. Based on the research, now I know why I was satisfied by nutritional density that had nothing to do with the amount of calories I was ingesting.

This is a new paradigm in nutritional science that, after enlisting in this program, forever changed my perceptions of the true meaning of true wellness. I now know it is not the amount of calories that matter in achieving a healthy lifestyle; it is the make-up of nutrition (nutritional density and composition) that is contained within the calories.

Phil, a friend of mine who lost almost 200 pounds, was astonished at the weight he released. Not only was he not hungry but he completely changed his eating habits because his cravings diminished almost overnight. This is not magic, it is really happening to tens of thousands of people.

Researchers and scientists are beginning to recognize the new paradigm for food, nutrition and wellness – it has to be about nutritional density and not calories. Stop counting calories and instead make every calorie count for your genes, immune system and most importantly for your quality of life.

That is why people are achieving extraordinary results on this nutritional fasting solution. Like my friend Mark who was full and satisfied even though he was eating a fraction of the calories he once thought he needed to survive when he was nearly 600 pounds.

No matter how many empty calories he consumed he still was not satisfied because those foods were devoid of all the 51 nutrients necessary to satisfy his body. Will power cannot work if you do not have the super calories that have the 51 nutrients. This nutritional fasting approach contains more than 51 of the essential nutrients and that is why Mark and I were not hungry along with so many others who have completed the nutritional fast.

Imagine a new gasoline additive were invented that allowed cars to get 100 or 200 miles per gallon instead of approximately 20 miles per gallon. This is the very same concept behind the nutritional super calorie. Just as the car would use much less gasoline and still travel much farther than before, this nutritional fasting approach provides the body with significantly more nutrients in much lesser amounts of calories. The body is able to function much more efficiently.

For me, the nutritional fasting approach was and is far and beyond a weight loss program. By introducing me to these extraordinarily dense foods, the nutritional fasting approach and the super nutritional calories they contain, I was catapulted into a lifestyle of extraordinary and maximum wellness.

I now have more energy, sharpened mental clarity and a new zest for life – benefits that were just as significant as the weight loss I achieved. Nutritional fasting has set me on a path toward youthful aging, longevity and a maximization of my personal human potential. I've achieved a state of well-being that keeps me energized and engaged constantly in my daily life. It allows me for the first time in my life to achieve two critical goals: first and foremost is to live healthier and longer. Second, I believe it is allowing me to maximize my human potential. My energy, mental clarity, lower stressed, boundless energy and sleeping like a baby each night are just a few of the benefits that have convinced me I am maximizing my human potential also.

How Would You Use More Energy in hour life?

This is why this program is so much more than a weight-loss strategy. I hear story after story about how people are getting so much more out of nutritional fasting than just the weight and most importantly the fat they are releasing. Recently, I got a call from a woman named Sharon who had been on the nutritional fast for six days and said she is amazed at the amount of energy she has and she can't believe how well she is sleeping. Although she wanted to lose weight she now says the energy and the deep sleep she gets far surpass the weight she is releasing.

My Personal Trainer Loves the TDOS Solution after Achieving Amazing Results

My own personal trainer told me just last week that he cannot believe how this has helped him reduce his overall body fat percentage, increased his flexibility and most importantly recovery time. This is a young man who is in incredible shape and has enhanced and improved his performance. Although he was skeptical at first, now he says this is the only protein and/or nutritional fasting program he will ever use and recommend to his clients. These stories are so common now that I have just included a few to give you an overall picture of what you might experience. After all, it is your experience on this nutritional fast and at the end of the day that is the most important aspect.

What Is a Super Food Shake Day?

A Super Food Shake day is very important part of the TDOS Solution's process that prepares the body to truly take advantage of the nutritional fasting days. My body began to burn fat even during the pre-fast period as I cut out unnecessary elements of my daily diet, such as caffeine, sugars, diet sodas and alcohol. I only drank a shake for breakfast and dinner and ate a healthy 400-600 calorie meal of my choice for lunch. This initially can be 2 to 5 days prior to do a nutritional fasting day.

During this time, I began consuming a minimum of eight 8-oz. glasses of water each day. In order to get the most out of my nutritional fasting experience, I drank half my body weight in number of ounces of water a day. Water is an integral part of any fasting program and drinking the necessary amount of water daily beyond fasting is an important habit to maintain smooth functioning within the body. This does not mean that water can be replaced with the small amounts contained in tea or soda. Pure water is the lifeblood of the body and a main vehicle for carrying nutrients. It also disposes of the body's waste and facilitates detoxifyification processes.

Every day through urination, perspiration and respiration, we lose the equivalent of at least eight 8-oz. glasses of water. In order to replenish this supply we must drink substantial amounts of clean, purified water.

Nutritional Fasting Days

After increasing my water intake and familiarizing my body with nutritional fasting nutrients during the Super Food Shake days, I began two days of nutritional fasting consecutively. In the TDOS Solution's approach, all nutritional fasting days are always the same; solid food is replaced with the aloe Vera, mineral enhanced liquid nutrition drink, whey protein mini meal snacks and a Super vitamin capsule.

In the first 24 hours of nutritional fasting, while solid food was not consumed, my body used up the sugar and glycogen stored in my liver and began producing growth hormone to trigger fat burning and support lean muscle mass.

On the first day of the nutritional fast, I consumed four ounces of the aloe vera nutrients four times a day, along with six to eight of the nutritional mini meals and two Super vitamin capsules. Because this nutrient dense food flooded my body with massive amounts of nutrients, vitamins and the "Mineral Suites", fats and proteins, I didn't experience hunger, even without solid foods.

Though the body begins its detoxification processes on the first nutritional fasting day; by the end of the second day, excess sugar and carbohydrates stored in the liver are used up and intense detoxification really is being achieved.

Within just the first 24 hours of nutritional fasting, the detoxification has started as the body burns excess glycogen (stored sugar in the liver) and during the second 24 hours it begins to detoxify by burning stored fat for energy. The very fat in which the impurities are stored. The body begins to detoxify as it burns off this excess fat (the glutathione in the shakes and the polysaccharides in the aloe attack the toxins and pull them apart and make them water soluble so they can safely be eliminated through the kidneys and the liver) and thus people lose pounds and inches quickly and safely. Throughout the nutritional fast, the body continues to increase levels of growth hormone to build muscle as the fat was released. People actually experience their body fat percentage decreasing as they continue to detoxify. This is a huge reason why world class athletes are now using nutritional fasting approaches. They are seeing reduction in fat and increase in lean muscle mass which improves their athletic performance, stamina and recovery time from work outs and injuries.

For me, the first two days of the nutritional fasting days really showed up in how well my tight jeans were fitting. Was this possible? In such a short period of time I was shrinking and I felt great with lots of energy.

After the first round of nutritional fasting days, I completed days of replenishment (super shake days which can be 5 or 7 days) so my body could rest and prepare for another round of serious nutritional fasting. By the morning of my next round of nutritional fasting, I was amazed at how much I was shrinking and how much energy I had. It astounded me that this nutritional fasting approach was already changing my world. After drinking half or nearly half of my body weight in number of ounces of water daily, I realized there was no way this weight loss could be explained away as just a loss of "water weight."

After those two days of Nutritional Fasting, I returned to a shake for breakfast, a single healthy meal at lunch and another shake for dinner along with a combination of super vitamins and snacks. The shakes provided the perfect combinations of carbohydrates, fats, proteins and Mineral Suites to continue the fat burning and nutritional fasting processes. I continued this routine through for another minimum of 5 to 7 days (this is up to you). I returned to a state of deep nutritional fasting after the Super Food Shake days were completed; my body resumed detoxifyifying and intense fat burning. These days were great opportunities for my body to really "clean house" of the more toxins so I could achieve maximum wellness and weight loss.

By following all recommendations in The T D O S Solution's nutritional fast, my body's functions continued efficiently and effectively, undisturbed by my major dietary changes.

I also have other friends who did the nutritional fast and said they had no weight to lose at all and they were shocked to drop pounds they did not think they had to lose. Of course, it was their bodies shedding this extraneous fat that was only there to store the impurities. As the body began to detoxify itself, it let go of this extra fat. That is why this nutritional fast has so many people scratching their heads and saying, "I cannot believe my scale." That is because they are used to conventional dieting, which simply does not and cannot produce such life-changing results in such a short time period safely. This is revolutionary and can, in fact, transform your beliefs about diet, exercise and your human potential.

Although results may vary, people are astounded at these seemingly average results. Still, many traditional dieters are excited if they can lose a pound a week. And by constantly replenishing any water flushed out of our bodies during the fast, this was guaranteed not to be a mere water weight loss that will be gained back right away. Knowing we could achieve our weight goals so quickly and safely motivated me and many other people to continue the program.

TDOS Solution's Your Race to Maintenance Approach

What do you do you finish the first phase (this can be a week or two, or a couple of months) of nutritional fasting if you have more weight to lose like Mark and myself? Or, you feel so good you want to nutritionally fast some more until you feel more satisfied?

Your Race to Maintenance Phase is Even Easier to Get to Your Goals

To provide the most effective means of long term weight loss success, Dr. Dennis Harper and I developed the "TDOS Solution's Your Race to Maintenance[1]" program because, for many who have just completed the beginning phase of nutritional fasting, their bodies risk abandoning full detoxification mode if they choose to immediately return to their old eating habits. Thousands have experienced a rapid completion to their goals. The schedule is an easy guide for you to follow until you reach your goal to begin maintenance.

A free TDOS Solution advisor is also available during this period to assist and ensure that the solution is followed correctly to achieve the best possible results. As the name implies, Your Race to Maintenance is to get you to a maintenance program safely with the least amount of effort in the shortest period of time possible. Your body will thank you and reward you with living healthier and longer.

---

1 For more information see Appendix III - Sample Chart: The TDOS Solution's Your Race to Maintenance.

Feast Days Include an Additional Meal at Dinner Time

To maintain the same detoxifying and the burning of fat after nutritional fasting, the body now requires more fuel. Unlike most conventional diets, this requires an increase in nutritionally dense calories while continuing to infuse the body with the massive amounts of vitamins, nutrients and the "Mineral Suites". "The T D O S Solution's Your Race to Maintenance" program can begins within a week or two of starting and continue for five days or more till you do another nutritional fasting day; I did it in 5 day increments (again you go at your own pace) by having a super shake for breakfast, a healthy lunch, a healthy dinner (you get to have dinner with your family or significant other) and a super shake for dessert. These five days we call "feast days" that include regular meals with the family as well as shakes. This makes it so much easier. Unlike a diet, this program actually increases the daily caloric intake with nutrient dense calories. These Feast Days are followed by two days of deep nutritional fasting for total 7-days the way I did it. I repeated this 7-day cycle for three consecutive weeks for a total 21 days. This is in addition to beginning the fasting solution for a little over a week that I did. I chose to do this put my body on a nutritional fast course for a full month. This is how I did it and this may not be the best way for you to start. There is not set in stone and you will find what works best for you. I am just sharing what I did 11 years ago. That is where a T D O S Advisor can be a great help to tailor a solution that works for you.

During the "T D O S Solution's Your Race to Maintenance" period, it is important that the shakes be the final meal of the day to supply the body with that special blend of enzymes, nutrients and trace minerals for continued fat burning. Since the amount of solid food is reduced on these days, the body's rate of fat burning and its basal metabolic rate – the rate at which calories are burned when the body is at rest – are slowed, and the individual may experience a plateau in weight loss. However, drinking the shake keeps carbohydrates down so they don't interfere with the human growth hormone production and will ensure sustained fat burning.

If you want to lose more weight do what works best for you. Your Race to Maintenance is up to how you do on your initial phase of the T D O S Solution's nutritional fast. Your Race to Maintenance nutritional fasting solution should be at your own pace. You can do it fast or a more gradual pace and most people find they still achieve incredible results in the long run no matter how they choose to do it.

Even with a lot of weight to lose, many people find they are able to maintain this T D O S Solution's nutritional fasting approach by utilizing Your Race to Maintenance until they reach their goals. As long as they are careful to consume calories comprised of no more than 40% carbohydrates and they eat no more than 600 calories per meal, their bodies are properly fueled to continue detoxify and burning fat. As they continue to feel better and become more nourished and active, the new life they are achieving motivates them throughout the process.

I spoke to a recent nutritional fasting participant in his mid-thirties who really had very little weight to lose. His name is Will and he only lost a few pounds, as that was all he needed to lose. He says, "I cannot believe the amount of energy that I have. It is not speed energy; it is natural and long lasting."

Another participant who is a sales manager in a high stress job said she is waking up at 6 a.m. and jumping out of bed. She said before the nutritional fast she dreaded mornings and now she has to make herself sleep in until 6 a.m. She is amazed that all day long she has energy and is not getting the cravings during the midday that she used to get. She says, "Many days I have to remind myself to eat lunch as I am so satisfied. You could have never convinced me there could be such an amazing food. It is wonderful to feel so full of energy and vitality."

My good friend Charlie started at 414 pounds and has released an astounding 42 pounds utilizing the Race to Maintenance program after his nutritional fasts. He cannot believe that he is not hungry. He failed on all the previous diets he tried because he always felt hungry. On Your Race to Maintenance he is able to stick to it. My other friend Fred who weighed nearly 400 pounds and who has lost almost 100 pounds also cannot believe that he has been able to stay on Your Race to Maintenance and it is changing his life. Whether you have 20 or 200 pounds to lose this can really work like nothing you have ever done before.

Personally, this was such a miracle for me. I was able to adhere to the TDOS Solution's Your Race to Maintenance requirements by following a list of recommended foods, fats and complex carbohydrates and the great variety of recipes included in this book kept me within the healthy 600-calorie range for meals. I was able to lose 30 pounds total by doing nutritional fasting for a short period of time and then switching to Your Race to Maintenance program. That changed my life forever. I would never look back nor do I ever want to go back to where I was!

TDOS Solution Advisors

The nutritional fast schedule and free advising services offered through this program were equally as important to my nutritional fasting success as the constant flow of nutrients. With encouragement and education, I was able to attain better results in both weight loss and overall health. As we said this is not one size fits all and the Advisors can assist in the best way to start and move you to Your Race to Maintenance at the best time so you can reach your goal of getting to maintenance as safely and quickly as possible.

If you like the authors of this book are not a nutraceutical chemist and need help in assembling this new nutritional approach we invite you to enlist the help of a TDOS Solution Advisor to guide you without charge. You are free to assemble all of these ingredients on your own as we have laid them out for you if you are so inclined.

For me, these advisors were invaluable to take out all the guesswork about how to properly access this new nutritional approach. They developed and sent me schedules and assisted with any concerns about nutritional fasting during my first few days of starting the nutritional fasting solution.

For people with any health challenges, the TDOS Solution advisors can modify the program accordingly to make it a better fit the individual. It is always recommended that anyone with health challenges check with their health professional or doctor before starting this nutritional fasting solution.

An overview of the Nutritional Fasting Solution

A Nutritional-Fasting Lifestyle to Maximize Your Wellness Potential

Here are the basics of what you do to begin—and continue until you have reached your goals, and then go on a simple maintenance program:

> **NOTE:** These are suggestions and general guidelines for you to follow as you see fit.

- The first few days: Do Super Shake Days for up to a week = Intermittent caloric reduction

- The next two days: Deep Nutritional Fasting Days = 48-hour nutritional fasting

- The next 5 to 7 days: Super Shake Days = Intermittent caloric restriction

- Followed by two days of Nutritional Fasting Days = 48 Hours nutritional fasting

- The next 5 to 7 days: Feast Days = Reduced caloric restriction

- Then two Days of Deep Nutritional Fasting Days = 48 hours nutritional fasting

- Repeat the 5 to 7 days of Feast Super Shake Days and two days of nutritional fasting until you reach your desired goals.

The terms "Super Shake," "Deep Nutritional Fasting" and "Feast" were explained above.

Sustaining the Nutritional Fasting Lifestyle

People ask me all the time, "Do I have to do this for the rest of my life?" My answer is always the same. It starts with a question and that question is, "Why wouldn't you want to fast every day?" Toxins don't go on vacation or mysteriously disappear from our world. In her book Detoxify or Die Sherry Rogers MD says that every time Glutathione goes out and hunts and pulls apart and renders a toxin harmless the Glutathione gives up its life. In other words for every molecule of a toxin that Glutathione destroys safely we lose one molecule of Glutathione as well. This would also make logical sense when it comes to the toxin hunters polysaccharides. If Glutathione and Polysaccharides are doing their job then we must continually everyday replace and replenish the depleted stocks of both as they continue to detoxify our bodies.

In other words if you do not continue to resupply the body with Glutathione (from Whey or the Vegan shakes) and Polysaccharides (from the inner heart gel of Aloe Vera) then you will severely reduce the body's natural ability to detoxify itself.

So I would ask this question instead.

Why wouldn't you want to continue to supply your body on a daily basis with the very molecules that give our bodies the natural ability to detoxify itself?

Toxins are entering us 24/7 365 days a year and they never take a day off.

The Human Body does not Store Protein

A more important reason for these whey protein shakes is that our bodies do not store proteins. Our bodies store fats and carbohydrates but we do not store protein. Chicken, fish, soy and many other forms of protein just do not have the levels of ingredients, including the amino acids and the added major minerals, micro minerals and Ultratrace elements the "Mineral Suites".

Also (other than mother's breast milk), these whey protein shakes from New Zealand are simply unsurpassed as a source of protein to reduce the risk of Sarcopenia (loss of muscle mass) and to supply your body with the nutrients that allow the body to continuing fasting. The scientists certainly agree that un-denatured whey protein on its own is so necessary for optimal health. With the addition of trace minerals and enzymes, the New Zealand shakes should include ingredients that are essential to the human body. It's no wonder so many people call them "super shakes."

Now you can probably see why just consuming a New Zealand super whey protein Shake each morning could give you so many advantages really over any other food you can possibly consume. It has so many benefits backed up by science that the real question you should ask yourself is why wouldn't I have a New Zealand super whey protein Shake every morning for breakfast. For me it comes down to one simple concept: I cannot find a better food to put into my body each morning that will give me the greatest chance to maximize my human potential.

Super Shakes from New Zealand at a Glance

In addition to containing superior protein, these shakes are unique for many reasons. Each "Super Shake" contains:

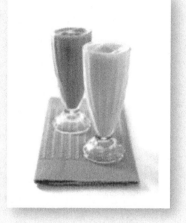

- New Zealand whey protein and milk protein from cows that are not injected with antibiotics or growth hormones.
- Un-denatured protein processed using low-temperature high-filtration pasteurization, as opposed to high heat pasteurization typically used in North America that greatly reduces the amino acids available to the human body.
- Proteins from cows in New Zealand that are fed grass not corn.
- Pre biotic fiber, primarily from flax seed and prebiotic fiber called isomaltooligosaccharides. Not all fiber is the same, and this prebiotic fiber in particular is so important to our bodies because it feeds healthy flora (good bacteria) and increases it in our digestive tract. This is beneficial to our overall health.
- Whey protein and milk protein with a similar ratio that is found in mother's breast milk, which is 60% whey protein and 40% milk protein.
- No artificial flavorings.

- No artificial sweeteners. Stevia is used as the sweetener (stevia contains no sugar and is naturally derived from the stevia plant). As a result, these shakes taste great yet they have a very low glycemic index.
- High content of good fats, including, olive oil, sunflower oil and coconut oil.
- No soy or soy-derived ingredientes.
- No genetically modified (GMO) ingredients.
- Extremely low lactose combined with lactase, which is an enzyme that aids in the digestion of lactose.
- Protease, an enzyme that helps to break down protein into particles called peptide that makes the protein much easier to absorb.
- Gluten and wheat free
- The Mineral Suites.
- The great thing is that you feel really satisfied because of the massive amount of nutrients contained within each shake. Remember, the key to satisfying our hunger is nutritional density, not how many calories we eat.

If you can find a more nutritious food than these super food shakes on this planet please let me know... so I can take it!

Maintenance and Plateaus

How do I maintain once I have gotten to my goals moving forward on a daily basis?

Every day, The TDOS Solution's easy maintenance program is recommended for maintaining weight and most importantly optimal health. I've accomplished this by consuming two ounces of the Aloe Vera juice enhanced with the "Mineral Suites" each morning, along with a New Zealand super whey protein Shake to sustain the levels of necessary nutrients, vitamins and "Mineral Suites" needed to maintain my fat-burning processes. I drink another two ounces of the aloe vera super juice before going to sleep to continuously assist natural detoxification of my body of everyday toxins and impurities. I also put my body through a two-day nutritional fast once every two months to rid it of those deeply embedded impurities trapped in fat cells.

Though it is important to continue to select from the list of recommended foods after completing the nutritional fast, it does not mean that "guilty pleasure" foods such as pizza, ice cream or alcohol cannot be enjoyed in a nutritional fasting lifestyle – as long as they are consumed in moderation.

After completing the TDOS Solution's nutritional fasting's approach and, if while on the maintenance approach you begin to experience food cravings again or become fatigued, overwhelmed or depressed, this could be a warning sign that the body has gone back into sugar-burning mode. Sugar burning mode is good for a very short period of time if you are going to run a 100-yard dash.

The body was meant to burn fat for long-term energy. In sugar burning mode you will constantly seek out sugars and carbs to replace the sugar that is rapidly used up. Fat burning produces much higher energy and much more long-term energy. The sooner you can get into and maintain fat burning the more energy you will have and the better you will feel. You can combat sugar burning by immediately completing just one nutritional fasting cycle to return your body to detoxifying mode to burn off toxic fat.

As is the case with traditional diets, it is possible to hit a plateau. These plateau periods may indicate that the body has slowed down or stopped detoxifying or too many simple carbohydrates, refined sugars or artificial sweeteners have been reintroduced into the diet to cause the body to enter starvation mode from the overconsumption of empty calories. Otherwise, the body may have achieved a state of equilibrium and will retain fluid for a period of time until a new equilibrium point is set, causing the body to dump the excess fluid. The key during any of these plateau periods is to not get discouraged, and to continue to self-motivate with the prospect of enhanced energy and full-rounded wellness.

Once individuals are familiar with what to expect on each day of any nutritional fasting program, exercise can enter into their daily routines. However, it is not recommended to start a nutritional fast and a new exercise program at the same time. When beginning this program, I was advised to walk a minimum of 30-60 minutes every day, preferably in the morning, to promote fat burning. Though I was told a 60-minute walk was ideal, if I could only walk for 15 minutes at a time, I walked twice a day for 15 minutes and then built myself up to 30 minutes. When it was available, I also jumped on a trampoline for 30 minutes as a great form of daily exercise.

By combining exercise and these nutrient-rich foods, my body was able to function efficiently by burning fat for energy. I cannot stress enough that this was not merely a weight loss program for me; weight loss was a side benefit of my newfound nutritional fasting lifestyle.

Adhering to the recommended regiment and consistently ingesting the rare combination of ingredients, allowed my body to detoxify itself naturally so I could accomplish long-term optimal health and wellness, extend my longevity and maximize my personal potential.

The recommendations set forth in the TDOS Solution's approach in this book are to help you achieve a nutritional fasting lifestyle. Recognize toxicity as the cause for systemic problems throughout the body and deal with the body as a whole to truly solve them. And although single-point solutions are helpful in specific applications, specific-point nutrients cannot deal with the systemic needs to maintain overall wellness of the body.

History has proven that new solutions and approaches are needed to update the belief systems and eliminate the common misconceptions about nutritional science. To thrive on this toxic planet, we must continue to educate ourselves on the potentially harmful effects of our surroundings and vow to make changes in our daily lifestyles. Nutritional fasting is a step toward reducing each of our own "toxic burdens" and ultimately sets us on the path toward long-term health.

Conclusion

Once in a great while something so extraordinary is discovered that it changes the world and your life if you choose to take advantage of it.

The toxic world we live in has been anxiously waiting for this life-changing discovery to be made.

This book has revealed this amazing discovery of nutritional fasting to you for the first time and made you aware of what is possible to live an extraordinary and healthier life.

Many of the scientists I have worked with are terrified at what is coming at us if we continue to do what we have been doing and expect a different result. That is the definition of insanity.

How will we cope with three babies born every day who will develop diabetes in their lifetime? There will not be enough insulin.

How will we cope with projections that say in 30 years 100% of America will be overweight?

Can we afford to do nothing?

Can you afford to continue to do what you have been doing?

Even if you are a purest who does not drink or smoke and only eats organic and exercises regularly? All of those things are still not enough if you are interested in living as long as you can and as healthy as you can.

Imagine that the number of people who will become sick in the very near future will overwhelm the ability of drugs, health professionals and hospitals to deal with this oncoming Tsunami of obesity and health-related problems. We are a "sick-care" world already and it is getting worse at an alarming rate. By the year 2112 it is estimated that nearly one million people will die of heart disease.

Some experts estimate that we now consume more than two trillion prescription drugs a year in North America. That represents nearly 50% of all the prescription drugs on planet earth. This is today; it is not what will be required in the future.

In addition, our water, air and food are becoming more and more hostile to our very existence. We build mountains of food that lasts a long time on the shelf but does very little to sustain us minute by minute, hour by hour, day by day and month by month. As a result, each year we lose a little bit more of our ability to maximize our human potential no matter what our age.

We have learned very well to live this less than healthy lifestyle by being overweight, devoid of energy and loaded with stress and brain fog; as if this is the way it has to be. How bad does it have to get before you do something better for your body?

This book offers great hope and a real solution to a fate that may come your way if you do what you are currently doing and ignore the overwhelming evidence that a drastic new approach is needed. You are not alone. Instead of joining the legions of the sick you can now become part of the healthy that are fit, trim and full of energy. Maximize your wellness and human potential and, most important-ly, to live healthier longer.

The nutritional fast is not a cure for anything. If the body is given dense nutrition it is capable of amazing things that I see every day of my life. If we give the body the proper fuel it simply functions better in all respects. As I said earlier, eat a low-quality form of protein and it takes your body several months to recover from the effects. There are simple things you can do that are pointed out in the book. It is not a pipe dream or some broken promise but rather the reality of a nutritional fasting lifestyle that is attainable once you make a choice to do it.

I realize that most of you are as skeptical as I was. That skepticism is only natural given the choices we have all made. Like most of you I had been disappointed over and over again with the next great breakthrough ("hope dope") in diet, health and nutrition only to discover that it was too good to be true and it left me broken-hearted and discouraged. And yet, when the next one came along I eagerly tried it thinking this might be the one. Does that sound familiar?

Is it any wonder you and I should be skeptical?

After many of these disappointing experiences I have found that the T D O S Solution approach is a major breakthrough in nutritional science and it is "the one." It is the real deal as they say. Never before, have so many people had consistent long term life-changing-results day after day month after month year after year. This is the first real long-term solution that can lead to a long-term healthy life.

Those who need to lose weight normally say "my scale must be broken" when they see dramatic weight loss typically in a very short period of time.

Those who do the nutritional fast because they like the idea of giving their cells an "oil change" often say "I really did not believe it was possible to feel this good. I have more energy than I ever have had I just feel wonderful."

Athletes are amazed at the improvement in their lean muscle mass, drastic improvements in their athletic performance and their quick recovery time after working out.

Remember what Dr. Ruggiero said food is the genetic information that we communicate to our genes. What kind of genetic information are your food choices communicating to your genes?

This nutritional fasting approach is not too good to be true; it is better than that. There are more than a million people who have done it safely with amazing results. And it is for everyone, whether you are an athlete, healthy, overweight or not.

I invite you to just give it a try and in turn it may change your life. Your best years can truly be ahead of you if you are willing to adopt a nutritional fasting life style now.

We realize you may still have questions before getting started, based on your own individual goals or maybe you just need more information. Our nutritional T D O S Solution Advisors are available to answer any and all of your questions and, if you do decide to join us, they will advise you through the nutritional fast for free.

People ask me all the time, "Do I have to do this forever?" I just smile and say, "When you think the toxins are going on vacation and when the toxins do then you can stop."

If you can find a better food to put into your body each day please tell me and I will eat it!

The most important concept I have repeated numerous times is that your real desire to do the nutritional fast is simple, "to live healthier for as long as you can." I don't know a single human being on this planet who is not interested in that.

I leave you to decide. As the famous scholar Hillel once said, "If I am not for myself, who will be for me?"

Results

Real people have seen real results with The T D O S Solution. This is what happened to me. My success gave me a reason to believe that this nutritional fasting approach was going to change my life, and it did.

Is it time for you to change your life now?

For more information, please feel free to contact us at: whydietsarefailingus.com

Bibliography

Acheson, K. et al. (2011). Protein choices targeting thermogenesis and metabolism. *The American Journal of Clinical Nutrition*, Vol. 93 No. 3 pp. 525-534.

Baillie-Hamilton, P. (2005). *Toxic Overload*. New York: Avery.

Beach, R. (1936). *Modern Miracle Men*. Washington, D.C.: U.S. Government Printing Office.

Campbell, W. et al. (2001). The recommended dietary allowance for protein may not be adequate for older people to maintain skeletal muscle. *Journal of Gerontology: Biological Sciences*, Vol. 56, Issue 6; pp. M373-M380.

Colgan, M. (2001). *The New Power Program: Protocols for Maximum Strength*. Apple Publishing Co.

Dangin, M. et al. (2001). The digestion rate of protein is an independent regulating factor of postprandial protein retention. *Am J Physiol Endocrinol Metab.*, Feb;280(2):E340-8.

Edwardes, C. (2003, September 14). Mr Banting's Old Diet Revolution. *The Telegraph*. London.

Encyclopædia Britannica. (2012). Retrieved July 30, 2012, from http://www.britannica.com/EBchecked/topic/90141/calorie

Enig, M. (1995). *Trans Fatty Acids in the Food Supply: A Comprehensive Report Covering 60 Years of Research.* Silver Spring, MD: Enig Associates, Inc.

Enig, M. (2000). *Know Your Fats : The Complete Primer for Understanding the Nutrition of Fats, Oils and Cholesterol.* Silver Spring, MD: Bethesda Press.

Enig, M.; Fallon, S. (1999). *Nourishing Traditions.* Washington, D.C.: New Trends Publishing.

Environmental Working Group. (2005, July 14). Study Finds Industrial Pollution Begins in the Womb. *News Release.* Washington, D.C.

EPA, U. (1990). *The National Human Adipose Tissue Survey.*

Fallon, S. (1996). Tripping Lightly Down the Prostaglandin Pathways. *Price-Pottenger Nutrition Foundation Health Journal,* 20:3:5-8.

Fallon, S. (2001). *Nourishing Traditions.* Washington, D.C.: New Trends Publishing.

Felton, C. et al. (1994). Dietary polyunsaturated fatty acids and compositions of human aortic plaque. *Lancet,* 344:1195-1196.

Finkelstein, E. (2012). Obesity and Severe Obesity Forecasts through 2030. *American Journal of Preventive Medicine,* Vol. 42, Issue 6, Pages 563-570.

Foxcroft, L. (2011). *Calories & Corsets: A History of Dieting Over 2000 Years.* London: Profile Books.

Gruber, B. (2002, May 25). *The History of Diets and Dieting.* Retrieved from CarbSmart: http://www.carbsmart.com/historydiets.html

Grun, F., & Blumberg, B. (2006). Environmental Obesogens: Organotins and Endocrine Disruption via Nuclear Receptor Signaling. *Endocrinology,* Vol. 147 No. 6 s50-s55.

Harper, D. (2012). Doctor of Osteopathy

Holtcamp, W. (2012). Obesogens: An Environmental Link to Obesity. *Environmental Health Perspective,* 120:a62-a68.

Houlihan, J., Kropp, T., Wiles, R., Gray, S., & Campbell, C. (2005). *Body Burden: The Pollution in Newborns.* Environmental Working Group.

Hyman, M. (2009). *The Ultra Mind Solution.* New York: Scribner.

Karnani, M. et al. (2011). Activation of Central Orexin/Hypocretin Neurons by Dietary Amino Acids. *Neuron,* 72: 616-629.

Kim,J; Li, Y; Watkins, B. (2011). Endocannabinoid signaling and energy metabolism: a target for dietary intervention. *Nutrition,* June 27 (6):624-32.

Lassek, W.; Gaulin, S. (2012). *Why Women Need Fat.* New York: Hudson Street Press.

Lasserre, M. et al. (1985). Effects of different dietary intake of essential fatty acids on C20:3 omega 6 and C20:4 omega 6 serum levels in human adults. *Lipids*, Apr;20(4):227-33.

Mann, T. et al. (2007, April). Medicare's Search for Effective Obesity Treatments: Diets Are Not the Answer. *American Psychologist*, pp. Vol. 62, No. 3, 220–233.

Miller, D. (2011). Retrieved from www.lewrockwell.com: http://www.lewrockwell.com/miller/miller38.1.html

National Institutes of Health. (2009, March 16). Study Helps Unravel Mysteries of Brain's Endocannabinoid System. U.S. Department of Health and Human Services.

Ogden, C.; Carroll, M. (2010). *Prevalence of Overweight, Obesity, and Extreme Obesity Among Adults: United States, Trends 1960–1962 Through 2007–2008*. Centers for Disease Control and Prevention.

Pennings, B. et al. (2011, May). Whey protein stimulates postprandial muscle protein accretion more effectively than do casein and casein hydrolysate in older men. *The American Journal of Clinical Nutrition*, pp. 93(5):997-1005.

Perrine, S. (2010). *The New American Diet*. Rodale Inc.

Peters, L. H. (1918). *Diet and Health: With Key to The Calories*. Chicago: The Reilly & Lee Co.

Pimentel, D. L. (1986). *Pesticides: Amounts Applied and Amounts Reaching Pests*. American Institute of Biological Sciences.

Pinckney, E. et al. (1973). *The Cholesterol Controversy.* Los Angeles: Sherbourne Press.

Pollan, M. (2006). *The Omnivore's Dilemma.* New York: The Penguin Press.

Schauss, M. (2008). *Achieving Victory Over a Toxic World.* Bloomington, IN: AuthorHouse.

Stitt, P. (1982). *Beating the Food Giants.* Natural Press.

STOP Obesity Alliance Research Team. (2010). *Improving Obesity Management in.* Washington, D.C.: The George Washington University School of Public Health and Health Services.

The Endocrine Society. (2009). *Endocrine-Disrupting Chemicals.* Chevy Chase, MD.

USDA. (2011). *Sugar and Sweeteners Outlook, No. (SSSM-273).* Washington, D.C.: U.S. Department of Agriculture.

Valero-Garrido, D. et al. (1990). Influence of Dietary Fat on the Lipid Composition of Perirenal Adipose Tissue in Rats. *Annals of Nutrition and Metabolism,* 34:327-332.

vom Saal, F. et al. (2012). The estrogenic endocrine disrupting chemical bisphenol A (BPA) and obesity. *Molecular and Cellular Endocrinology,* 354: 74-84.

Weinberg, B., & Bealer, B. (2001). *The World of Caffeine: The Science and Culture of the World's Most Popular Drug.* New York: Routledge.

Wilkinson, A. (1995, June 5). Oh, What A Tangled Web. *The New Yorker*, p. 34.

Wilson, L. (2011). *Selenium: A Critical Mineral for Health and Healing.* Prescott, AZ: Center for Development.

Appendix I _____

18 Reasons to Try The TDOS Solution Approach

1. **Liver Support** ... the liver is the main detoxifying organ of the body. It takes fat-soluble toxins so that they can be excreted in the urine. This is made easier with the amino acids in the products recommended in this book.

2. **Antioxidant Protection** ... free radicals damage cells. Antioxidants are substances that fight free radicals.

3. **Aids in the Loss of Weight** ... it's proven that weight loss decreases the chances of diabetes, cancer and heart disease thus increasing your life expectancy.

4. **Enhanced Mental Abilities** ... a recent study showed that mental abilities improve with weight loss. Many TDOS Solution users report weight loss as a benefit.

5. **Increased Energy** ... do you want to feel better and accomplish more? The TDOS Solution isn't an "energy drink," but rather delivers a level of nutrition that will help you get more done each day without feeling like you have been overworked.

6. **Immune Support** ... nutritional fasting and removing impurities from the body while replenishing it with vital nutrients can improve immune function and lessen immunity threats within the body.

7. **Better Cellular Function** ... our cells need essential nutrients and compounds to be healthy and communicate. Nutritional Fasting delivers such nutrients and creates an environment where cells can effectively communicate and perform.

8. **Premature-Aging Protection** ... nutrient deficiencies, impurities and toxins can damage our cells and organs and lead to premature aging. Nutritional Fasting slows the onslaught of the toxic world and creates a shield of protection for increased energy and a sense of overall rejuvenation.

9. **Better Digestion** ... The T D O S Solution products delivers enzymes and other vital nutrients for the digestive tract. The digestive system is replenished with good bacteria and enzymes to help with the breakdown and absorption of food.

10. **Enhanced Nutrition** ... the best way to take control of your health is through improved nutrition. One of the few things in life that you can control is: you get to decide what goes into your body - and what goes into your body determines what type of body you will have. T D O S Solution offers a terrific new nutritional approach.

11. **Weight Control** ... it's no secret that obesity is a huge problem in today's society. Many degenerative diseases are associated with obesity, either as the cause or a complicating factor.

Nutritional Fasting may help support the loss of excess fat and water and increase muscle mass.

12. **Fights Obesity** ... obesity is on the rise and has been rising since 1985 when the CDC (Center for Disease Control and Prevention) started to monitor obesity. It is now estimated that almost 26% of the adult population is obese or morbidly obese. Nutritional Fasting as part of a healthy lifestyle can reduce the likelihood of obesity.

13. **Adaptogenic Support** ... some of the T D O S Solution approaches contain adaptogens, which have been used by Olympic athletes for years. Adaptogens are agents (usually botanicals) that help the body "adapt" to physical and mental stress.

14. **Less Cravings** ... as you nutritionally fast it's very common to have cravings for unhealthy foods go away. These cravings are replaced with a sense of wellbeing and satiety.

15. **An "Aura" of Wellness** ... want to look good and have that air of good health and energy? It's almost impossible to do this if you're not eating nutritionally dense foods like those from The T D O S Solution.

16. **Youthful Skin** ... skin cannot be healthy without the proper nutrition from the inside. This also applies for impurities in the body. Nutritional Fasting and replenishing your body with vital nutrients can lead to smooth, youthful-looking skin.

17. **Rejuvenation with Mineral Suites** ... The T D O S Solution approach contains vitamins, nutrients and major minerals, micro minerals and Ultratrace elements which are the key to a healthy body. Cells cannot function properly without them. Minerals and Ultratrace elements are easily absorbed and, once in the body, speed up innumerable cellular reactions.

18. **Gastrointestinal Support** ... replacing poor-quality, low-fiber foods with high-quality, nutritionally dense foods can improve digestion and enhance gastrointestinal function

Appendix II _____

Recipes for Your Success

You are not alone and this is why we have put together some wonderful recipes to get you started.

These recipes have been carefully put together to give you plenty of choices. The following recipes and vegetarian alternatives are recommended as lunch options to be eaten during the program or as a delicious and healthy meal anytime. All the recipes include acceptable and suggested foods to integrate into your diet if you choose to partake in the T D O S Solution nutritional fast and begin your personal journey to full wellness. Enjoy!

Radical Red Potato Salad

1 cup red potato– cut into bite size pieces

1 cup chicken broth (low sodium, so you control the seasoning)

1 cup water

1 tsp. sea salt

1 tbsp. white wine vinegar

2 hard-boiled eggs

1 stalk celery

1 tbsp. parsley

¼ cup chopped red onion

½ cup steamed broccoli

Simmer potatoes in the above brine mixture of chicken broth, water, salt and vinegar for 15 minutes on medium low and then boil on high for 2 minutes to reduce the liquid. Drain the potatoes reserving ⅛ cup of the liquid. Place potatoes in a serving bowl.

Dressing:

⅛ cup of reserved potato liquid

⅛ cup olive oil

1 tsp. white wine vinegar

1 tsp. Dijon mustard

⅛ cup of the cooked potatoes (optional)

Blend the above dressing mixture together (the addition of cooked potatoes thickens the dressing a bit). Pour the dressing over the potatoes in the bowl. Then add the chopped celery, parsley and red onion. Mix and toss. Season with salt and pepper. Serve at room temperature with steamed broccoli on the side.

Quinoa Pilaf with Swiss Chard, Toasted Pine Nuts

1 cup quinoa

2 cups vegetable or mushroom broth

3 tbsp. pine nuts

¼ cup sun dried tomatoes

1 tbsp. olive oil

2 cups uncooked Swiss chard

1 clove garlic, chopped

¼ cup garbanzo beans (chick peas)

½ tsp. paprika

½ pepper

¼ tsp. sea salt

In saucepan, put in 1 cup quinoa, 2 cups broth, salt, pepper, and paprika. Bring to a boil. Immediately turn down heat and let simmer for 10-15 min. While quinoa is cooking, heat ½ tbsp. olive oil on low heat in skillet and add pine nuts. Toast for 2 min, watching carefully not to overcook them. When nuts are lightly browned, add the other ½ tbsp. olive oil and garlic. Add Swiss chard and sauté for just a moment until wilted. Toss the nuts, Swiss chard and sun-dried tomatoes into quinoa. Feel free to experiment with substitutions, as this can be a creative dish. The broth both flavors the quinoa nicely and also adds good minerals.

Fiesta Black Beans and Rice with Green Salad

½ cup dried black beans

2 strips kombu (seaweed)

½ cup uncooked brown rice

1 cup water

1 yellow onion

2 cups mixed greens

½ tsp. cumin

½ tsp. chili powder

1 clove garlic

Juice from 1 lime

½ tsp. sea salt

¼ cup fresh cilantro

1 small fresh tomato

The night before you wish to have this dish, soak the black beans in water. Drain the following day. Cook on low or in a crock pot with fresh water the next day with seaweed strips, yellow onion and salt for a couple hours or until tender. In a saucepan, combine cooked brown rice, cumin, chili powder, garlic and salt with 1 cup water. Bring to a boil, then immediately reduce heat and simmer for 10-15 minutes. Lay the mixed greens on a plate and pour the brown rice and black beans on top. Squeeze limejuice from over the top and garnish with cilantro and fresh tomato.

Harvest Roasted and Stuffed Butternut Squash

1 medium butternut squash, halved and seeded

1 clove garlic, minced

1 cup cooked barley (hulled or hulless)

½ tsp. sea salt

½ tsp. pepper

½ tsp. sage

½ tsp. rosemary

1 tsp. olive oil

½ thyme

1 carrot

½ cup mushrooms

2 tbsp. walnuts, chopped

Preheat oven to 400 degrees. Place squash in foil and put into a baking dish with olive oil and bake until tender, approximately 50 minutes. Cook barley with sea salt (with a ratio of 2:1 water to barley) for about 45 minutes. In a skillet, sauté garlic, carrots, mushrooms with sage, rosemary, thyme and pepper. Combine vegetable mixture with barley and stir in walnuts, mixing well. Divide barley and vegetable mixture between the two halves of the butternut squash.

Carrot coconut and Ginger Bisque and Baby Butter Lettuce Salad

Bisque:

2 tsp. coconut oil

1 medium onion, chopped

3 tbsp. finely chopped fresh ginger root

3 cups carrots, chopped

1 medium potato, peeled and chopped

8 cups vegetable stock

1 can coconut milk (13 ounces)

Fresh parsley or cilantro, chopped (optional)

Heat the coconut oil in a large pot. Add the onion and ginger and sauté just until the onion is translucent. Add the carrots, potato and vegetable stock. Bring to a boil, cover, reduce heat and boil gently until the vegetables are tender, about 30-45 minutes. Purée the soup in batches in a blender or food processor. Add salt to taste and gently swirl in coconut milk. Serve plain or garnished with chopped fresh parsley or cilantro.

Salad:

1 small head of baby butter lettuce

1 slice red onion

½ avocado

Toasted shaved almonds

½ fresh mango, sliced

Spicy citrus dressing:

Juice of 1 lemon

2 tbsp. chopped shallots

2 tbsp. white wine vinegar

¾ cup extra-virgin olive oil

Pinch of cayenne

2 pinches of both salt and pepper

Wash and shred the butter lettuce. Top with sliced red onion, bite-sized avocado, toasted almond and fresh mango slices. Toss in the spicy citrus dressing. This salad accents the bisque by using mango to complement the coconut and also adds the warmth of ginger and cayenne to support digestion.

Miso Soup with Ginger and Root Veggies

3 cups vegetable stock

1tsp. miso paste

1 tbsp. dried wakame (or any seaweed, i.e. nori, kombu)

1 cup chopped kale

½ lb. shitake or portabella mushrooms

⅛ yellow onion, sliced

1 carrot peeled and chopped

1 celeriac root (celery root) peeled and chopped

1 tbsp. chopped ginger

2 cloves garlic, chopped

¼ cup uncooked quinoa

Pour stock into pot or large sauté pan. Add seaweed and simmer for 5 minutes. Add onion, carrot and other veggies. Sauté for 2 minutes. Add ginger, kale and shitake mushrooms and sauté for 3 minutes. Add garlic and uncooked quinoa and simmer for 15 minutes. Remove from heat and add miso paste that's been mixed with a little water or broth. Do not boil miso; it will kill the beneficial enzymes.

Golden Lentil and Sweet Potato Stew

½ cup dry yellow lentils

¾ cup chopped sweet potato

1 tbsp. ghee (clarified butter)

½ yellow onion

1 large carrot, chopped

1 clove garlic, minced

1 large celery stalk, chopped

¼ cup fresh parsley, chopped

½ tsp. sea salt

½ tsp. pepper

½ tsp. onion powder

½ tsp. garam masala

2 cups water

3 leaves of spinach chopped

Put 2 cups of water and lentils into small pot with chopped sweet potato and salt and bring to a boil. Immediately lower heat and let simmer 30 minutes. While lentils are cooking, sauté garlic, onion, carrot, and celery in olive oil. When lentils are cooked add vegetable mixture, pepper, onion powder and garam masala. Simmer for another 15 minutes. Add spinach greens for just a minute. When cooking is complete stir in fresh parsley and salt to taste. This is a great recipe to use up extra veggies. It is easy to heat up and very filling.

Miso Sesame Roasted Tempeh and Cauliflower with Spinach

3- 4 ounces tempeh

1 cup cauliflower

1 tbsp. miso paste

1 tbsp. rice wine vinegar

¼ cup water or vegetable broth

2 tbsp. sesame oil

1 tbsp. coconut oil

2 - 3 cups spinach, packed

Dash of Siracha (optional)

2 tsp. black sesame seeds

Cut the tempeh into triangles. In a small bowl, whisk together miso, rice wine vinegar, water or broth until the mixture is a thin paste. Thin it out with water or broth if necessary. Toss the tempeh and cauliflower in paste until gently coated. Sprinkle with black sesame seeds. Place in a baking dish in the oven on 350° for about 10-15 minutes.

In a skillet briefly sauté spinach in coconut oil until barely wilted. Finish with a dash of sesame oil, optional Siracha and a sprinkle of sea salt. Serve the tempeh and cauliflower on a bed of spinach for a delicious and easy meal.

Spinach and Goat Cheese Frittata

1 garlic clove

1 zucchini

1 small shallot

2 eggs

1½ cups chopped spinach

1 tbsp. butter

1 small red bell pepper, chopped

½ tsp. sea salt

½ black pepper

½ cup chopped mushrooms

3 cherry tomatoes

½ tsp. red pepper flakes (optional)

¼ cup goat cheese

Preheat oven to 350 degrees. Sauté garlic, onion and pepper in butter. When almost cooked, add in zucchini, mushrooms and spinach; cook until spinach is slightly wilted. In separate bowl, whisk together eggs, salt, pepper and red pepper flakes. Add vegetables and stir in goat cheese crumbles and chopped cherry tomatoes. Pour mixture into small cake pan that has been greased and bake for 30 minutes. Let frittata cool for about 5 minutes before serving.

Roasted Acorn Squash with Mushroom Gravy and Green Beans

1 small acorn squash

2 cups sliced mushrooms (shitake, portabella, chanterelle, oyster, etc.)

1–2 tsp. miso paste

2 cloves garlic

¼ cup onion

¼ tsp. umboshi plum vinegar

¼ cup nutritional yeast (available in health food stores)

sea salt to taste

½ to 1 cup water

⅛ cup olive oil

1 cup fresh green beans

2 tsp. slivered almonds

Cut the acorn squash in half and scoop out the seeds. Place the squash on a baking sheet and bake at 350 degrees for about 30 minutes or until soft to the touch. In a skillet, sauté garlic and onion in olive oil until transparent and aromatic. Add mushrooms and let them cook down until soft, add water as needed. Add the water, nutritional yeast, vinegar and sea salt to taste. Simmer until well-cooked down. Remove from heat and add miso paste that has been blended with a little water. Steam the green beans until bright green and still a bit crunchy. Scoop out the insides of the squash and arrange green beans on top. Pour the mushroom mixture over squash and steamed green beans and top with slivered almonds. This is a delicious and nutritionally dense meal.

Roasted Fennel and Veggies in a Balsamic Glaze

½ onion, sliced in chunks

1 parsnip

½ cup chopped red, green and/or yellow bell peppers cut in large chunks

½ fennel root cut in chunks

3-4 of garlic cloves peeled (leave them whole or halve them)

1½ tbsp. olive oil

1 tbsp. balsamic vinegar

½ cup course corn meal

¼ tsp. sea salt (or to taste)

Roast Vegetables:

Place fennel and veggies in a large open baking dish and toss generously with olive oil and balsamic vinegar, salt and pepper to taste. Roast at 350 degrees for about 30 minutes.

Polenta:

Bring 1 cup water or low-sodium chicken broth to a boil. Reduce to a simmer. Pour in corn meal steadily, stirring constantly. Cover and cook on low heat for 40 – 50 minutes, stirring every 10 minutes or so until polenta is thickened. It should come away from sides of the pan and be able to support a spoon. Pour polenta onto a wooden cutting board to cool once it is solid, let stand for a few minutes. Serve with roasted vegetables.

Turnip Puff with Seared Rainbow Chard

Turnips are a delicious root vegetable that are super high in minerals, vitamin C and folic acid. Feel free to use green chard in place of rainbow chard.

1 small turnip, cubed	Pinch of sea salt or tamari
2 tbsp. ghee (clarified butter)	generous sprinkle of pepper
2 eggs, beaten	¼ cup dry breadcrumbs
2 tsp. potato starch	1 bundle of rainbow chard, de-
1 tsp. maple syrup	stemmed and torn into bite size pieces
1 tsp. baking powder	1 tsp. coconut oil

Cook the turnip in salted water until tender. Combine turnip, ghee and eggs. Mix dry ingredients together and add to the turnip mixture. Put into a greased casserole dish (7" x 11" works well). Combine melted butter and crumbs. Sprinkle on top. Bake 25 minutes at 375 degrees.

In a sauté pan heat 1 tsp. of coconut oil, add the rainbow chard, sea salt or tamari and leave for about one minute until wilted. Serve hot over the turnip puff.

Sunshine Raw Vegetarian Nori Rolls

Instead of rice, this recipe uses sunflower seeds that are much richer in protein, fiber and good fat making this meal balanced and protein dense unlike most veggie nori rolls. They are easy to make and, once you get the hang of it, you can experiment with the inside ingredients as you get comfortable with the process.

½ cups hulled sunflower seeds

½ mango sliced into long strips

2 green onions, green parts only, chopped and divided

2 tbsp. limejuice

2 tbsp. tamari

1 clove garlic

3 small collard green leaves

3 sheets nori

1 cucumber, peeled, seeded, and cut into strips

1 avocado, halved and thinly sliced

Soak the sunflower seeds in cold filtered water for a couple of hours. Place the soaked seeds into the food processor with the tamari, garlic, limejuice and half the green onions. Blend into a smooth paste. Place the nori sheets flat on a cutting board, line with one leaf of collard greens. Spread about 2 tbsp. of sunflower paste onto collards (a spatula works well). Then down one side stack the cucumber, avocado, mango and remaining green onion so it makes a line from top to bottom. Roll the strips up until tight as you can and dab some water along the edge to seal. Cut into 1 inch pieces and serve. Dip in tamari if you like and enjoy,

Heirloom Gazpacho, Spanish Quinoa and Avocado Salad

This is a delicious recipe especially in season when you can get some plump juicy garden tomatoes. The quinoa substitution for the rice is a great way to up the protein and the whole thing finished off with a dollop of avocado salad is just perfect.

Gazpacho:

3 pounds ripe heirloom tomatoes

1 clove garlic

2 tsp. salt

4 tbsp. olive oil

2 tbsp. good quality wine vinegar

½ green pepper (Italian, long thin)

2 cucumbers

½ small onion

1 cup water

Optional garnish to serve on top of soup:

½ small onion chopped

½ green pepper chopped

½ cucumber chopped

1 small tomato chopped

Place heirloom tomatoes in the blender until they are pureed. Strain to take away the skin and seeds. Put the remainder of the ingredients into the blender with the tomato puree, garlic, salt, cucumber, onion and pepper. Process until pureed, with the motor running, add the oil in a slow stream and then add the vinegar.

The mixture will thicken and change color as the oil emulsifies. Stir in the water. Chill until serving time. If the soup is too thick, stir in more tomato juice or water. Garnish with any of the optional suggestions.

Spanish Quinoa:

1 cup cooked quinoa

½ cup small onion, chopped

½ cup medium green pepper, chopped

1 tbsp. butter

4 ounces tomato sauce or diced tomatoes

2 mild green chilies (optional)

¼ tsp. sea salt

Simmer the onion, pepper, green chili, and sea salt together in butter in a hot skillet until cooked and soft. Toss into cooked quinoa and stir in tomato sauce.

Avocado Salad:

1 avocado

½ cup cucumber, chopped

¼ cup fresh red onion, chopped (optional)

¼ cup cilantro, chopped

juice from half a lime

sea salt to taste

Coarsely chop the cucumber and avocado. Finely chop the onion and cilantro. Mix gently into a bowl to keep the avocado from mashing. Sprinkle with limejuice and sea salt.

Roasted Fig and Goat Cheese Salad

This is a delicious salad for a light meal. It has both chevre and sprouted pumpkin seeds for protein. Sprouted seeds are more nutrient dense than un-sprouted seeds, so if you can find them it is worth it, or you can sprout your own.

⅓ cup apple cider vinegar

1 tbsp. molasses

2 tsp. extra virgin olive oil

2 tbsp. sea salt

4 large fresh figs cut in half

1 – 2 handfuls of organic greens

2 oz. chevre (soft goat cheese)

Course ground black pepper

¼ cup sprouted pumpkin seeds

Combine first 4 ingredients in a medium bowl, stirring with a whisk. Add figs and toss to coat. Remove figs with a slotted spoon, reserving vinegar mixture.

Place figs in a cast-iron or ovenproof skillet. Bake at 425 degrees for 8 to 10 minutes. Remove figs from pan and place on a plate. Immediately add reserved vinegar mixture to the hot pan, scraping pan to loosen browned bits. Pour into a small bowl. Let figs and vinaigrette cool to room temperature.

Place salad greens on a platter. Arrange figs over greens and sprinkle with chevre and pepper. Gently mix in sprouted pumpkin seeds. Drizzle with cooled vinaigrette.

Tortilla Espanola and Arugula Salad

Tortilla Espanola or Spanish omelet is the most commonly served dish in Spain. This single-serving recipe can be increased proportionally to accommodate a large party or enough for leftovers.

Tortilla:

1-2 eggs, beaten

Salt to taste

1-2 tbsp. olive oil

1 small red potatoes (lower glycemic), peeled and thinly sliced

1 onion, peeled and finely chopped

green olives, chopped for garnish

Heat olive oil in a frying pan. If you are making one serving, a very small pan is best. Add the potato and fry for a couple of minutes until it starts to turn golden. Add the onion and mix together in the frying pan. Meanwhile, crack the egg(s) into a bowl and whisk with a bit of salt. When the potato and onion are golden brown add the egg(s). Make sure the potato and onions are fully covered by the eggs. Fry this gently on low heat for 3-4 minutes. While it is cooking, free the sides and the bottom with a spatula so it is easier to remove. Once it is lightly browned on the bottom, place a plate upside down over the frying pan.

With one hand on the frying pan handle and the other on top of the plate to hold it steady; quickly turn the frying pan over and the omelet will fall onto the plate. If you want to fry the other side, place the frying pan back on the range and put just enough oil to cover the bottom and sides of the pan. Let the pan warm for 30 seconds or so. Then slide the omelet back into the frying pan. Use the spatula to shape the sides of the omelet. Let the omelet cook for 3-4 minutes. Turn the heat off and let the tortilla sit in the pan for 2 minutes. Turn the pan over and place the tortilla on a serving plate. Let it settle for about 5 to 7 minutes before serving. Garnish with green olives, which is a Spanish tradition. It is also delicious with tomato sauce.

Salad:

2 cups arugula, washed and chopped

¼ cup tomato, chopped

1 tbsp. flax oil

squeeze from ½ a lemon

sea salt to taste

Mix together the arugula and the fresh tomatoes. Drizzle with flax oil, lemon and salt to taste. Serve alongside the tortilla.

Sneak Preview

The TDOS Syndrome

Foreword

I believe the content presented in Peter Greenlaw's latest book, The TDOS Syndrome™, is both visionary as well as revolutionary. Visionary, because it gives a bird's eye view of some of the most significant issues threatening our individual health and how those issues interact with each other synergistically. This has repercussions for our society's ability to survive into the future. Revolutionary, because it approaches our problems with a new perspective that is completely different from any current recommendations about what it takes to remain healthy.

As Americans, life and our standard of living are facing some tough challenges. We are on the threshold of a frightening reality. Our population is aging; as the population bulge of the Baby Boom snakes through the life cycle, with 10,000 Boomers retiring every day. With the increasing needs of this aging population, personal and financial support is being called forth from subsequent generations, who will have to provide for this sector through their contributions. The financial burden is daunting. The difficulty arises due to the discrepancy between the large numbers of Boomers versus the smaller populations of the generations that follow. In addition, we are in a frightening escalation of several significant health trends.

Healthcare costs have spiraled out of control. The current dialogue in Washington between both political parties is unhealthy. The rhetoric of a "slowdown" of the rate of rise in healthcare costs, as projected by the supporters of the Affordable Care Act, completely ignores the fact that, as a population, some of the toughest battles with regard to our health as a nation have only recently begun to be understood.

Our healthcare system is focused on treating disease once it manifests. This increases treatment costs. We treat osteoporosis or high blood pressure once they develop. We treat Type II diabetes with oral medications and only marginally approach "real" lifestyle, diet and exercise changes. We treat high cholesterol with expensive and not entirely risk-free statin drugs. We address sleep apnea with uncomfortable oxygen masks or surgery. We perform expensive and risky surgeries on our morbidly obese patients. These examples point to how medicine is practiced in the United States today; it is predominantly reactive. That is, we wait for disease to manifest and then we intervene with pharmaceuticals, surgery or other procedures. While necessary and not entirely avoidable, it is time that we begin to approach our health, or lack thereof, in a much more proactive, pre-emptive, personal and individual manner.

Peter Greenlaw's book highlights four cofactors that, together, are magnifying the downward spiral of our health. The culprits are toxins, nutritional deficiency, overweight and stress: The TDOS Syndrome™.

Toxins: Our bodies face an increasing toxic burden of harmful chemicals that assault us everywhere; in the air we breathe, the water we drink and the food we consume. We are regularly exposed to a chemical cocktail of roughly 80,000 substances. Only a few have ever been tested regarding their long-term effects on human health. Our understanding of their interactions with our bodies is at best incomplete. A flurry of information is coming to light about the toxicity of some of these chemicals. The picture it paints is potentially grim, a frightening canvas that depicts the future of the human species.

Chemicals like Bisphenol A and even the commonly used weed killer Glyphosate, which finds extensive use in modern agricultural practices, are potent endocrine disruptors. The chemicals affect our endocrine system, which functions in close concert with our reproductive system, affecting the hormonal systems and the fertility of our adult population. What is even more frightening is that they can and will have an influence on the immature, developing systems of our children at an early age, when their bodies are most prone to programming errors that will affect them for the rest of their lives. These toxic chemicals potentially affect our ability to procreate. Such an impact imperils the survival of the human species on this planet.

Nutritional Deficiency: The standard nutritional recommendations from physicians, dieticians, clinical nutritionists and other health professionals are: consume a well-balanced, diversified diet of carbohydrates, proteins and fats, with focus on fruits and vegetables and healthy fats and oils. They recommend limiting red meats, processed foods and simple sugars. It's challenging to maintain a healthy diet. Meanwhile we are bombarded by well-intended advice along with sales pitches and distorted opinions and recommendations from special interest groups in our industrialized food production system.

The industrial food industry mass-produces cheap food with a long shelf life to feed an ever-growing global population. In my opinion, the quality of the foods we consume has steadily declined. Little nutrition remains. After reading the following pages in The T D O S Syndrome™, you will have a better understanding of this discrepancy. The paradox: We are a nation that is overfed but sadly undernourished. As the author poignantly observes, "Food will never be enough by itself," certainly rings true for me in my own study of this topic. We need to look at food as not only providing us with needed macronutrients—carbohydrates, fats and proteins—and thus the calories (just like gasoline that keeps the engine running)—but also in terms of the overall content of micronutrients.

Micronutrients are the crucial vitamins, trace minerals phytonutrients, enzymes and so on. Today we see the steep decline in micronutrients in our raw food, a century in the making. The unknowing consumer is not informed about the lack of nutrients in our food. The food companies obfuscate these facts and blur the truth to maintain the status quo. An interesting study published in 2009 illustrates this point. The incidence of multiple micronutrient deficiencies is more prevalent in overweight and obese adults, as well as children. In other words, those dietary habits that lead to excess weight gain also predispose the individual to have nutrient deficiencies! When you add a calorie-reduction diet on top of the micronutrient deficiency and overall nutritional deficiency of raw food products, it is no wonder that typical diets fail. Even focusing on the so-called healthy foods isn't sufficient. Nutrients are depleted even there. Our bodies simply cannot sustain functioning with a further nutrient shortage.

Another interesting recent study points to a link between weight loss diets and an actual increase in blood levels of toxins and also between diabetes and blood levels of toxins. This supports the author's hypothesis that toxicity, nutrient deficiencies and being overweight are directly interlinked.

Overweight: This poses another huge threat to our society as a whole. As a population, we are growing. I mean that in the literal sense. The percentage of extremely overweight people is at an all-time high. Our children and even our babies are fatter and in worse physical shape than they have ever been. Where, on the continuum from overweight to obesity, do long-term ill-health effects begin? While it depends on the individual, there is no question; financially devastating chronic diseases appear in those suffering from excess weight problems at a higher incidence.

Some of the common problems that I see nearly every day in my medical practice include heart disease, high blood pressure, diabetes, gastrointestinal reflux, sleep apnea, cancer, back pain and injuries, inflammatory diseases and more. These cause tremendous personal hardships for the individuals but also place a huge financial burden on our country. It will, in my opinion, become absolutely unsustainable and threaten to bankrupt our nation. Current estimates project that the annual expenditures associated with obesity-related diseases will grow from a current $150-170 billion to a projected $500 billion or more by the year 2030!

These are annual costs with the potential to increase exponentially, adding to our national debt. We can try to rein in our costs as much as we want through legislation. Until we get serious about the underlying root cause of these expenses (and our health), we will fail miserably, both as individuals as well as a society.

Stress: A favorite buzzword, stress forces us to run from crisis to crisis and to put out one fire after another with little reprieve for refueling and replenishing in between. We all know stress is bad and that we need to avoid it as much as possible. That is easier said than done. While we may have some degree of control over external causes of stress, most of us don't understand what stress does internally. Many have heard about the links to heart disease, high blood pressure and anxiety. Many people overeat because of stress. The problem runs much deeper than that. The factors described above, along with the constant assault of chronic excess stress which puts our body in a constant defensive and repair mode, creates a vicious vortex of self-perpetuating processes which insidiously accelerate our aging process and make us sicker faster.

Most of us are bombarded with advice on lifestyle, diet and exercise. Yet, despite all of this information available to us, the sad truth is that most of us will falter and succumb along the road. Mr. Greenlaw and his co-authors have a wonderful ability to break the problems down with a novel perspective, and then to reassemble them, showing the interconnections that make sense out of the bigger picture.

The TDOS Solution™, flows from this one into a solution that is both systematic as well as realistically attainable by each and every one of us. The choice of whether to continue with the status quo, or not, is up to us. The government, well intended as it may be and our current healthcare system are ill equipped to affect the changes at the scale called for.

I challenge you, the reader, to read the information contained in this book, to really understand the magnitude of the problem. Reading first about the syndrome and then about the solution, you will be amazed at the transformation that you are about to experience.

Dr. Bernard Lauder, M.D.

Born in Germany, Dr. Bernard Lauder, M.D., attended Germany's Gymnasium. He immigrated to the United States in 1976 on a gymnastics scholarship. He attended Western Michigan University, pre-med, from 1976-1980. He attended medical school at the University of Texas at Galveston from 1981-1985. At the University of Colorado, he served his residency as OB/GYN from 1985-1987. In addition, he went on to serve a residency in Anesthesia from 1987 to 1990. He is a diplomat of the American Board of Anesthesiology and has maintained a private practice in Denver in anesthesia since 1990. His special interests include physiology, especially as it relates to diet, metabolic syndrome, obesity inflammation, and exercise in general. He currently co-owns two gyms together with his sons.

DISCLAIMER: The opinions expressed are those of Bernard Lauber MD. None of these statements have been evaluated by the FDA. This book is for educational purposes only to make you aware of what is available through our research in writing this book and you decide if this information can help you to maximize your Wellness Potential.

It is believed by many doctors, researchers and scientists to be making us fat, tired, stressed out and generally preventing us from maximizing our wellness potential as well as our human potential.

The TDOS Syndrome is not a disease or an illness. And it is always recommended to consult with your medical doctor or health professional before embarking on any new diet, nutritional approach, solution or exercise regimen.

The New Health Conversation

TDOS

The Syndrome and Solution

The New Health Conversation Series

Peter GREENLAW

with

Drew GREENLAW

Nicholas MESSINA MD

Overview

The TDOS™ Syndrome and the TDOS™ Solution

In *The TDOS™ Syndrome and Solution*, we demonstrated that our nation is facing a health crisis. Almost no one is free from the effects of this crisis we now all face, which I call the TDOS™ Syndrome and Solution.

The TDOS™ Syndrome is composed of four interconnected cofactors: Toxicity, Nutritional Deficiency (or nutritional insufficiency), Being Overweight and Stress. I say that these are interconnected because each one feeds and intensifies the effects of the other three.

When it comes to maximizing our wellness potential traditional ways of thinking about health and medicine simply do not work all of the time what we need is a new approach, one that I call the TDOS™ Syndrome and Solution.

Nicholas Messina, M.D., says, "Since I was a boy I dreamed of becoming a doctor to help others and to make a difference. I realized my dream and began the practice of medicine with optimism and enthusiasm. Over the years, it became apparent that the more I helped people, the more help they needed. I began to feel that my best efforts were not making a profound difference. Over the past several years, by utilizing the TDOS Solution, I have empowered people to help themselves; which has caused a lasting change in their health and quality of life. This has been one of the most rewarding experiences of my medical career."

If Dr. Messina feels this passionately about the Solution, then certainly it's worthy of your consideration too.

TDOS Solution™ Preface
By Jerry Katzman MD

I am honored to have been asked to participate in not only writing a chapter within this book but to write the preface to it. Professionally, it is not only a privilege to know, Peter Greenlaw but it is with great pride admiration and respect that I have for him as a person and friend. It is strikingly evident in this book Peter's, determination, perseverance, insight, passion and conviction in trying to save the world one person at a time. He is the consummate researcher's researcher having read over 600 books by the world's leading experts on the subject of nutrition, diet, exercise, toxicity, obesity and new innovative technologies, including the world's leading geneticists, nutritional formulators and life coaches. He has traveled all over the world and given over 1200 lectures worldwide. He has interviewed hundreds of consummate professionals as well as everyday people from virtually all walks of life including children who suffer or have suffered with weight challenges, mental and progressive disorders. These disorders include an inability to concentrate or maintain focus, experience deep bouts of melancholy or manic behavior ,uneasiness, and/or cardiovascular symptoms and digestive symptoms i.e. headache, palpitations, blurry vision, fluctuating blood sugar issues etc. He has on a personal level experienced many of these challenges himself with a near death experience due to his own weight related, issues and consequences on his cardiovascular and digestive health systems. In addition he was plagued dealing with the crisis of his son Colin who suffered from paranoid thoughts, panic and maintenance of his focus and concentration. His own story and story of his family is at the core of his motivation and journey.

Peter as an investigator is like an expanding sponge. He continues to absorb as much as is possible all targeted towards his goal of bettering mankind and saving the world one person at a time. Unexpectedly, he is not a physician and yet has a grasp and perspective of the normal physiology and pathology of the body overall and unlike anyone that I have ever met in medicine including physicians and non-physicians alike today. This is so because you cannot find what he is teaching as being taught in Medical Schools (at least not yet) especially the T D O S Syndrome, the Solution and Why Diets Are All Failing Us.

Most importantly it should be noted that the opinions he espouses are not his opinions at all but the opinions of hundreds of authors and world experts (the greatest minds collectively) on various subjects uncovered through his incredible research. The key to Peter's success is his unrelenting thirst for knowledge and his need to give back to society and change the world. A Dedication that has led him to miraculously "connect the dots" and unfold the real story behind weight loss, diet exercise, nutrition and various related diseases.

So why did Peter chose me to write this preface? I believe because our stories are different and yet the same in many respects. We both believe we were brought together through divine intervention. A conclusion easily reached since the chances of us meeting were virtually impossible and off the charts and which I will explain.

I have been a practicing ophthalmologist and entrepreneur living in Tampa for over 25 years. Peter was from Colorado. My personal research had led me to discover the power of silver specifically the new technology silver. I was involved in a project to save the world by ridding it of Malaria through the use of the unknown benefits of Silver with Gordon Pederson M.D. PHD who I consider the world's leading expert on the benefits of Silver. In fact Gordon collaborated with me on the chapter in this book on Silver. I had been promoting the benefits of Silver when I was introduced to Peter through his interest in my preoccupation with the benefits of silver. We spoke and discussed our projects. Convinced that we were both going to change the world I became interested in why diets fail and he in silver. During my discussions with peter I explained that I had been healthy most of my life although admittedly, I had dealt with weight challenges since 10 years of age. I had been on every diet imaginable. The Scarsdale diet, St. Josephs Diet, nutra-system, weight watchers, south beach, Perricone diet, Atkins, etc. You name it I had been on it. In fact I lost weight on all of them; at least that is what I thought.

At 59 years old, I woke up suddenly with palpitations. I immediately went to a cardiologist which is even a scarier experience when you are a physician. My blood pressure was over 200/110. The cardiologist immediately placed me on water pills and medications and proceeded to draw my blood. An analysis demonstrated that my blood sugar was elevated, hga1c elevated, cholesterol elevated etc. I had routinely tested my blood, had normal exams my whole life, so this was not good. In fact I was heading into what is called Metabolic

Syndrome. A disorder with many bad side effects that could challenge my overall health and I was very concerned.

My doctor placed me on large doses of medications. It took over three months to get under "control" using the medications given to me by my doctor. Truthfully, I felt miserable. It was depressing and expensive costing well over and above what the insurance company would pay.

Then along came Peter and a preview copy of this book. When I received it, I immediately read it in one sitting. I was so excited I had to call Peter on the phone and told him that I thought he had "white bread" meaning he had something that would really change the world in concept if it worked. To me it made sense to work so I immediately embarked on the T D O S Solution's nutritional approach. The rest of the story is history.

I lost over 100 lbs. without diet, exercise or starvation safely and in a relatively short period of time. There is no question in my doctor's mind that the profound loss in weight enabled me to get off of all my medications. My blood sugar, blood pressure and cholesterol were all below normal. This again according to my doctor was due to the dramatic weight loss.

Let me state unequivocally as a medical doctor that in no way am I saying that the T D O S Solution was a cure for my medical problems and it is clear to me and my doctor that my improved health was due to the weight loss which I will be forever grateful for.

As a physician I would always advise you to check with your own health professional or doctor before embarking on any new diet or nutritional approach such as the T D O S Solutions approaches.

Well without sounding like an infomercial the next phase of my story began. So many people noticed my weight loss, I was continually asked what I did to lose so much weight and how did I do it.

To save my voice and free up my time dominated by my story, I decided to create a blog internet radio show talking about my experience and Peter so people would hear the story and read the book themselves. Then an incredible thing occurred. I ran the internet show of my blog story for approximately thirteen weeks when I received an email from a Web Based talk radio show in Chicago as part of the Tower group. I was advised that a patient had referred them to me and asked me if I would be interested in being a radio talk show host! While I had been on T.V., lectured and done radio interviews in the past, I had no experience as a talk show host. I accepted the challenge.

The show enabled me to interview the world's greatest scientists, physicians, inventors, technologies, technologists, patients and interesting personalities. Suddenly my life had completely changed. After seven months, my show became rated as number one on google! It was also picked up by iTunes, stitcher radio, etc. The show has now become my new passion and provides me with an ability to tell my story and Peter's story and to join Peter's mission of changing the world one person at a time. Through the radio show and the openness of working with peter I have been able to give back even more than my service as an ophthalmologist by collaborating and debating on approaches to many issues facing the world in health and advanced technology today.

Peter's inspiration has led me to the discovery of a multi-dose preservative free medication vial, the discovery of which has led now to the development of a preservative free vaccine. The vaccine will change the world by removing toxins from the vaccine where were previously tainted with preservatives which are implicated as one of the major causes of autism. Who would think that a non-physician researcher could change the world one person at a time? He has my vote! Peter has changed my life forever and I am forever proud, humbled and challenged by my association and friendship with such a world crusader. But what it is about this solution that is so special, different and enlightening, I will now explain. What if you didn't know what you always thought you knew and what if everything you knew was all wrong? Now you will finally know the truth as you read below.

Firstly, most of us by now have probably all heard about T D O S Syndrome™ in one form or another. Most people have heard of the terms Toxicity, nutritional Deficiency, being Overweight and Stressed out. We have heard it on T.V. the radio, magazines, newspapers, books, etc. So what is the secret sauce over this T D O S syndrome and T D O S Syndrome and the Solution? It starts with the coining of all four of these co-factors into a Syndrome because they are all very intimately interrelated. In addition it is the very nutritional approaches and solutions in this book that provides us with a solution NOW. It also takes into account that the solutions provided are forever evolving and being updated and will undoubtedly become part of future extensions of the same solution as science progresses. This book therefore is a work in progress as much as it is a masterpiece setting forth new principals and algorhythms to explain normal physiological processes of the body which we thought we knew as many were all ineffective or incorrect.

In Medical School physicians learn very little concerning nutrition and even less about vitamins, minerals, trace minerals and cellular cofactors. In truth we learn close to nothing concerning the interaction of our bodies and toxins on a cellular level when our bodies are overloaded by toxins. It is this gross lack of understanding and education which has left a gaping hole in the hull of the ship and led to principles and guidelines based on speculation and financial considerations not facts. The very foundation we thought we trusted has blinded us from understanding and being able to model how the body processes its foods, toxins assimilates or eliminates them as the case may be. Clearly the old health conversation of diet and exercise is based on a faulty premise and incomplete knowledge of nutrition and waste management of our bodies.

In a breath of fresh air on the subject it is in this book that a new revelation and set of principals are developed.

Without stealing Peter's thunder from this book I will just say that toxins are all around us. We get them in the air we breathe, the water we drink as well as the food we eat. We know the air is contaminated with jet fuel, industrial waste, etc. Our waterways are contaminated with industrial waste dumping, discarded drugs and chemicals and our foods contain antibiotics, herbicides, pesticides and GMO's. We learn in Medical school simply that all toxins are cleared from our kidneys and liver and eliminated in the urine and stool. However what is never addressed is what happens to the excess toxins when the body's kidneys and liver are overrun with toxins and cannot handle their excess. That is where the story of T D O S begins. We now learn that when presented with toxins the liver will start to package these toxins and store them into specialized fat cells known as "obesogens".

Once created these fat cells are difficult if not almost impossible to remove especially using the old health conversation techniques of diet and exercise we have all been taught. We know now that these obesogen fat cells have to be able to be converted to a water soluble form allowing the toxin to be released into the blood stream while at the same time allowing the toxin to be captured by a "toxin hunter" substance. Again this is not taught in any medical school and is novel to the T D O S Solution approaches and solution's contained within this book.

We know that when we starve we cause our brains to crave food. It also causes our fats to mobilize from our fat stores while releasing fats and fat products into the blood stream as well as stripping our muscle tissue to create sugar from proteins and amino acids. These fats are broken down further into ketones, FFA, toxins, etc. These fat byproducts are dangerous if accumulated within the blood stream and must be monitored by expensive blood tests and urine tests. At high levels they can cause seizure disorders and acidosis, etc. At the same time the brain senses that you are starving and burns more fat and muscle to create energy.

Eventually, in order to conserve energy, it shuts down your metabolism, and slows it down in order to hold on to your fats and muscle tissue and eliminate excessive muscle and fat stores from being lost. I mentioned earlier that T D O S Syndrome is intimately interrelated. Well here is how and again the new revelation in this book If you decrease the state of toxicity within one's body by providing the body with all the vitamins, botanicals, nutrients, major minerals, micro minerals, Ultratrace elements and co-factors that it needs, you can shut down the bodies central command directing muscle mass loss and wasting without shutting off the needed process of mobilizing fats and toxin release and a metabolism shut down or slowing. In addition will eliminate the brains desire to crave and be hungry. This is the perfect storm needed to allow you to control the weight loss process without starving but simply through an understanding of the normal physiology of the body now that the whole story is available to understand. With the system of breaking down fats uninhibited and the body's intense desire to crave and eat food turned off the body is in the perfect place to begin purging itself of toxins stored within the obesogens and other fat cells. There are however limiting factors in order to understand the process further. The body only produces naturally a small amount of a toxin hunter substance known as glutathione. Which again I am sure you may have heard of. However the production of Glutathione is woefully inadequate to eliminate the tremendous amount of toxins unleashed by the fat shedding toxin eliminating solution process. Therefore there is a need for some other toxin hunter substance to assist the body in the removal of toxins. Again as learned within the T D O S Solution you will become aware of these additional toxin hunting molecules and substances and how to use them. But simply to understand that once they are bound to the toxins they are eliminated in the urine and out through the liver.

In fact the fat cell unable to reuptake the toxins which have become bound and trapped to the toxin hunter's substances literally vaporize. As a result tremendous weight loss is manifest due to Fat loss not the typical muscle wasting known as" Sarcopenia" that we see on T.V. with stretched skin hanging low etc. and which is normally one of the consequence of diets.

While I have tried to simply touch on the principals of T D O S Solution within this book it is clear that we are able to do so because Peter has redefined what we do know because what if everything we thought we knew we didn't know and what if everything we knew was all wrong has come to pass and is true. We now know the answer. There is no doubt that you will be fascinated with the concepts, principles, knowledge and information shared by Peter in this book not to mention that it may be life changing for you too.

Enjoy!

Dr. Katzman emphasizes that it is always recommended to contact your health professional or physician before beginning any new diet, or exercise program.

Brief Bio

Born Bronx N.Y.

Graduated Boston University 1974 Bio-Medical Engineering

Graduated Medical School June 1980 Universidad Autonoma de Guadalajara, Jalisco Mexico M.D. degree

NY state 5th pathway clerkship in association with Albert Einstein College Hospital System-Providing One year of free clinical service to N.Y. State in an impoverished and underserved area of N.Y. (fort Apache in the Bronx)

Medical Internship-(Internal Medicine) 1981-82 Albert Einstein College Hospital System-Bronx Lebanon Hospital Center, Bronx N.Y. (fort Apache)

Residency-(Ophthalmology)1982-1985 Albert Einstein College Hospital System- Bronx Lebanon Hospital Center Bronx, N.Y.

Established the Dept. of Ophthalmology in Multispecialty Group Practice Brandon Florida July 1985-July 1986

Entered Private practice as an Ophthalmologist and Eye Surgeon- specialty anterior segment (cataract, corneal transplants, lasik, refractive surgery) 1986-2010

Made in the USA
Coppell, TX
02 January 2020